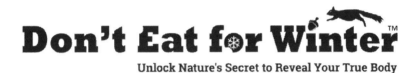

Don't Eat for Winter™

Unlock Nature's Secret to Reveal Your True Body

Cian Foley B.Sc., P.G. Dip.

IUKL Amateur World Kettlebell Champion

Edition 1: Published 2017
by UpTheDeise Enterprises,
Waterford, Ireland.

Printed Edition ISBN: 978-0-9554755-5-9
Kindle Edition ISBN: 978-0-9554755-6-6

Disclaimer: while every precaution has been taken in the preparation of this book, the publisher and author assume no responsibility for errors or omissions, or for damages resulting from the use of the information contained herein.

Results from applying the information contained in this book may vary between individuals, as there are many variables that affect weight, including, but not limited to, genetics, environment, metabolism, food intake, age, levels of activity and many other factors, which means results will vary also.

The statements contained within this book have not been evaluated by any medical or government health organisation. All content in this book is presented for informational purposes only. It is not intended in any way as a substitute for professional advice, diagnosis or treatment of any medical condition. Before undertaking any new health care regime, always seek the advice of your doctor, or other qualified healthcare professional, with any queries you may have regarding a medical condition and/or treatment of same. Under no circumstances should you disregard professional medical advice or delay seeking it because of the information presented herein.

www.donteatforwinter.com

Preface

I wrote this book to help others like me. If you are overweight and struggling to lose it, I wrote it for you in particular, but the information within is useful for most people, whether you want to start towards losing a lot of weight or finish your journey through losing those last few pounds.

Having been obese myself for over a decade, I know what it's like to live in a state of constant self-criticism, torturous denial, and to feel like I was trapped in a body in which I did not belong.

Where did I go wrong? Was it my fault? It made me miserable, and I felt worthless a lot of the time. I fooled myself and couldn't help binge eating, no matter how many times I tried to use my willpower to stop. I felt bad that I wasn't strong enough to fight these urges. I couldn't help myself, no matter how much I wanted to be a normal, healthy weight. I didn't realise I was the victim of powerful, natural instincts, and potent fat-depositing survival abilities, and an industry that preys upon them.

I now know that it wasn't entirely *my* fault, and if you're overweight, it isn't entirely *yours* either. We are products of both nature and our environment, and let's face it, our environment isn't natural anymore.

Nature gave us powerful instincts in order to survive and, in the western world, we have ingeniously overcome food shortages, but we haven't overcome our instincts to gorge. Therefore, we are caught in a conundrum that leans heavily towards chronic weight gain.

There *is* an easy way out and it took me years to figure it out; and believe me, I tried lots and lots of diets. I've found that this way of eating is manageable for me and has given me terrific results. I can't see why it wouldn't do the same for you too, as we are all on the same spectrum when it comes to energy and nutritional requirements. Yes, we are all slightly different, but we are fundamentally the same, otherwise breast milk wouldn't be so similar the world over – nature's formula for giving us the best chance at the start of our lives.

The diet (for want of a better word) is not a low- or zero-carbohydrate (or carb for short) diet. At its essence, it is a *controlled carb* diet, because carbs are primarily an instant energy food (especially refined sugary carbs). If your body gets an excessive amount of this energy supply, in particular, it will trigger processes to facilitate storage of all excess energy as fat for later use. In addition, these types of foods trigger instincts that make you want to gorge, which compounds the problem. Try eating just one or two fries in a fast-food restaurant, or just one piece of chocolate, and you'll find out how powerful these instincts can be, even if you weren't hungry in the first place.

Don't Eat for Winter outlines a way of eating, whereby you'll be satisfied with your food; you'll get plenty of natural carbs, protein, fat, vitamins and minerals to give you enough energy to see you through the day; and you'll get enough nutrients to keep your body in tip-top working order, while allowing it time to burn fat. In this way, you get the body nature intended you to have.

I am doing things now that I didn't think possible a mere five years ago. At 40, I'm running up mountains; benching 100 kilograms for reps at 78 kilograms body weight; doing pistol squats and handstand push-ups; winning kettlebell competitions, running for miles and miles without effort – and all the time, people tell me I look fantastic. I have abs (abdominal muscles) again, and great muscle tone, good skin, no pain, and lots of energy. I've heard many people complaining about aging, but I feel like I am defying it, and I can out-work many people half my age. This might sound arrogant, but it's not arrogance: it's a testament to the diet and, of course, the accompanying exercise that I do, which used to be a chore, but is now something I really look forward to. I think more clearly, sleep better, and feel unwell far less often.

I want to help you to feel this way too. I want you to become the hunter version of yourself – to take the form that nature intended for you.

Your DNA, through your cells, will create a completely new version of you within a couple of years, if you give it the correct input. The predominant input you can give them is food, so you must think carefully about giving the correct inputs to the most important asset you have: your body. Obviously, we need good air, water and sunlight too, but it is food that builds this biological flesh and bone machine of ours and makes us what we are. You literally are what you eat, and within two years you could be a completely upgraded model of yourself. You can start that journey tomorrow if you want to: it just takes a bit of knowledge about the types of things to eat, when to eat them, and the reasons behind these decisions.

I'm not saying you can't party and have fun and eat treats. I am that guy who overdoes it at parties, and I do overindulge now and again. But, you need to understand that this behaviour will have side-effects and may set you back a little. However, if you stick to the guidelines of the concept 80 per cent of the time, I am confident you will achieve great results, like I did. It's worth a try at least, and you won't be hungry. In fact, you will begin seeking out amazing, natural foods once you take note of how you feel, and the side-effects of eating them.

Thank you for choosing to read my book. I am rooting for you and I genuinely wish you the best. I want you to become the ultimate version of *you*.

It would make me very happy if the information in this book were to help you out even a little; and should you wish to share your journey with me and other friendly like-minded people, please consider submitting your success story using the following link:

www.donteatforwinter.com/testimonials

Acknowledgements

There are many people I wish to thank for the support they gave me during the preparation of this book.

First and foremost, I thank my wife, Nicola, for her patience with my time and grumpy moods because of all the late nights I spent writing. I thank her for listening to me ramble on about the various ideas and at the same time keeping an interested look on her face. I'd also like to thank her for being a guinea pig and becoming even more stunning at 40 than she was at 30 (if that were possible). She now weighs less than she did at 18, and has great muscle tone too!

I'd like to thank my good friends Kieran O'Sullivan, David Burke and Dr Mark Rowe, for being such positive influences in my life, and for setting me on the path that led me to my transformation and eventually, to the writing of this book.

Sincere thanks must also go the people who read various drafts of the book, including Kieran O'Sullivan, Keith Griffin, Emer Croke, Dave O'Leary, my wife Nicola, and my father Declan Foley, for giving such valuable feedback on its content.

I'd also like to thank Rachel Finnegan of Irish Academic Editing for her meticulous copy-editing, which has greatly enhanced the quality of the book and Lee Grace for producing the vectorised version of my logo. Thanks also to Anton Krieger for the use of the kettlebell photographs taken at the IUKL World Championships held in Dublin in 2015.

Finally, I'd like to thank you for purchasing and reading my book, which I genuinely hope will help you on your journey.

To my two lovely children, Siân and Daniel

Hopefully the world will be a much healthier place for you to live when you get to my age

Foreword

Dr Mark Rowe MB BCH BAO MICGP DPDDCH LFOM

'Don't Eat For Winter' is a novel way of thinking about the foods we choose to eat or don't eat each and every day of our lives. Truth is nowadays there is a tsunami of obesity and associated chronic health conditions from diabetes and dementia to coronary heart disease and cancer.

Now more than ever, the foods we are eating are increasingly coming under the microscope as we seek to understand the 'why', and we don't have to look very far because people are eating more sugar-rich and processed foods than ever before. Recent estimates put annual sugar consumption at a staggering 150 pounds+ per person (compared a mere 5 pounds per person in the 1700s).

The human body quite simply can't cope with this deluge of sugar and processed foods; the consequences are all around us. Therefore, I endorse this book for two reasons. Firstly because it encourages us all to look at our dietary habits through new eyes and understand that the food we eat has a significant impact on our health and wellbeing. Not just what we eat but understanding the when and the why. Perhaps more importantly for me the second reason - the author Cian Foley. I have known Cian for many years and he has attended several events I have hosted on health and wellbeing. His ongoing personal transformation over that time from couch potato to kettle bell champion has been nothing short of inspirational.

Here's the thing. You can be just like Cian too. Each and every one of us has that possibility of becoming more of a leader in our own wellbeing and make the steady sustainable changes that, over time, can add up to significant results in our lives.

Actions always speak louder than words and by his actions Cian is offering a new approach. It's working for him, perhaps it might work for you too! Good luck on your own journey of wellbeing.

Dr. Mark Rowe is a highly qualified and experienced medical doctor, author, speaker and a thought leader in areas of health, wellbeing and happiness. He is both founder and medical director at Waterford Health Park, an internationally acclaimed, award-winning healthcare centre. He is also author of 'A Prescription for Happiness' and 'The Men's Health Book' and an international keynote speaker on topics such as 'Wellbeing', 'Health Leadership', 'Generative Space' and 'Happiness'. Above all of this, he is a wonderful friend and role-model.

Table of Contents

List of Tables/Figures

Chapter 1

Don't Eat for Winter

(At least not all of the time …)

The fact that autumnal foods are so readily available all year around, creates a recipe for perpetual weight gain in order to prepare us for a winter that never comes!

Don't Eat for Winter

Once upon a Time …

… a long, long time ago, in a forest that used to exist nearby, people lived in a dangerous habitat with no supermarkets, no convenience stores, no international transport systems and no artificial preservatives. In this wild world, they could only eat what was available to them, as provided by mother nature on a day-to-day basis.

In spring and summer, they hunted and foraged, and ate mostly wild game, eggs, fish and seafood, along with whatever edible plants they could get their hands on. Autumn was a magical time, however, as everything became plentiful. Trees bore fruit, crops ripened, vegetables grew plump and so they feasted during the harvest and made delicious meals with their regular foods. They ate and ate until their bellies got nice and plump and their bodies became big and strong.

Then the cold, bleak winter set in, and as food became scarce and began to rot, they became very hungry and so very, very cold. Luckily, they were strong from the autumn feast, and their hardy bodies kept them warm and gave them enough energy to get through the worst of the winter months. When the spring came around again, their big tummies had disappeared like magic, and so they began exploring and hunting again most efficiently, and they lived happily ever after …

… until the following winter!

This is Where the Fairy Tale Begins …

Unfortunately, we are the ones living in a fairy tale, an artificial world that has diverged from nature. In this world, all of the seasons' produce are available to us all year long. It is we who need to break out of the magic spell from under which we are held, and realise that our bodies evolved in a prehistoric world: a world where the food provided by nature was designed to work with our bodies, in order to give us just the right amount of sustenance needed to survive the immediate future.

Nature provided staple foods such as meat, poultry, fish and eggs to give us the nutrients and energy required for our daily needs for most of the year. The seasons, particularly autumn, produced different types of foods such as fruits, vegetables (henceforth abbreviated to "veg"), grains, tubers, nuts and seeds, to prepare us for the seasonal challenges that lay immediately ahead.

With this in mind, consider the following statement:

Foods that ripen in Autumn are designed, by nature, to facilitate fat storage, in order to give humans and animals their best chance at surviving the food shortages, and cold, of winter.

It sounds obvious, right? So why is nobody saying it?

Survival of the ~~Fittest~~ Fattest

Getting fat is a talent! In the animal kingdom, there are many examples of creatures, such as squirrels, that gain weight during autumn. Many animals even hibernate during the coldest, most barren months of winter in order to survive it. Although human beings do not hibernate, we evolved in the same ecosystems as these animals, and no matter how much we try to separate from, and subdue, nature, we are still very much connected to it; and we still have very powerful instincts that overwhelm us and influence our actions, overriding our better judgement, from time to time.

Traditionally, we relied on nature's produce as and when it ripened; so it stands to reason that our physiology would have been affected by, and adapted to, the timings of this produce in similar ways to other mammals.

We are the product of evolution, and large pockets of our species would have been whittled down in parts of the world where the seasons were pronounced and winters were severe. In order to survive these bleak winters, which were periodic spells of food shortage/famine, and extreme cold, we would have relied on our fat reserves to assist our survival. It is logical, therefore, to suggest that those who were more efficient at storing fat, especially in these parts of the world, had a better chance of survival during those times. I would argue that this is the primary reason why many of us can put on weight so quickly and easily.

In evolutionary terms, this is an example of "survival of the fittest". However, *fit* in this instance means *fat*, so it really was a case of "survival of the fattest!"

Fat, of course, is an excellent, efficient, energy-storage system for human beings, and is also an insulator for the body, keeping the heat in and the cold out. Therefore, humans that were prone to putting on weight were more likely to last longer without food and in addition, they were also protected more from the cold. Scientists studying a 19.2 km open water swimming race in Perth, Western Australia, concluded that: "Increased BMI appears to be protective against hypothermia …" (Brannigan et al., 2015, p. 14).

Those who couldn't put on weight were more likely to die of starvation or hypothermia, or survived by adapting in other ingenious ways.

If you have a tendency to put on weight, don't beat yourself up, it is totally natural and is a talent you are blessed with by nature. You are a perfect product of nature and were born to survive weeks to months of famine and cold weather. Fortunately, and unfortunately, society has found ways of making the foods that nature provides available all year round, but some of these foods are designed to encourage us to store fat for winter, and so having them available to us all the time fosters indefinite weight gain.

Mother Nature: The Ultimate Moderator

The major problem nowadays is that we have supermarkets with every type of seasonal food available every single day of the year. Just walk into any one of them and you will see foods traditionally only available in autumn ever present. This is both a blessing and a curse: a blessing because we have a wonderful array of nutritious foods available to us whenever we want them, and a curse because our bodies and instincts have not yet adapted to cope with this new, abundant environment yet (and maybe never will, and do we want them to?).

Whenever a species cannot adapt to a new environment, it suffers, ie large portions of the population that cannot deal with the environment are whittled down. We are seeing this today, as chronic obesity – and related health issues such as heart disease, stroke, hypertension, some cancers and type 2 diabetes – has become one of the major causes of ill health within the human population, and it's worsening at an alarming rate. The global burden of disease study, 1990–2010, published in a special edition of *The Lancet* (Ezzati et al., 2012–1213, p. 2095), was reported on by *The Telegraph*, and suggested that eating too much is now a more serious risk to the health of populations than eating poorly, killing three times as many as malnutrition. According to Dr Majid Ezzati, one of the lead authors of the report, "We have gone from a world 20 years ago where people weren't getting enough to eat to a world now where too much food and unhealthy food – even in developing countries – is making us sick" (Adams, 2012, para. 4).

Of course, modern medicine can help to prevent people getting ill and prolong lives but this is akin to putting a sticking plaster over the problem: it doesn't address the underlying issue, which is that we eat too much of the wrong types of food.

Adams reports: "they believe being obese has risen from the 10th most important risk factor for death in 1990, to the sixth. More than three million now die from having a 'high body mass index', an 82 per cent increase" (para. 12).

There is obviously something fundamentally wrong with the way we eat, and this is causing untold hardship for our species. But, we do have a choice:

1. **Do we continue to adapt to this artificial environment?** Sacrificing the health of people who can put on weight easily, people potentially encoded with genes that were programmed to survive over the course of hundreds of thousands of years?

or

2. **Do we address the underlying issues and fix the problem?** Take a real look at what our bodies are capable of consuming safely, and educate ourselves about how to look after our most important asset, our body?

Do we have to go through all of this pain and suffering, or can we use our intelligence to eat within the parameters that we evolved to cope with?

I think that we have had our fun and it's about time we grew up as a species and took some personal responsibility for ourselves and our families, friends, and communities.

Piling on weight over weeks, months, and years, indefinitely, was never the intention of nature. Nature used to moderate the types of food we could eat based on whatever was "in season", and gave us the perfect balance of foods required for our survival at any given moment in time. Without this natural moderation, weight gain has become chronic and poses serious health risks, including type 2 diabetes, hypertension (abnormally high blood pressure) and heart disease, as well as creating all sorts of other physical problems and self-esteem issues. It's just not natural how we eat these days, and the bottom line is this:

The fact that *autumnal foods* are so readily available *all year around* creates a recipe for *perpetual weight gain*, in order to prepare us for a *winter that never comes*!

Thrifty Genes

I wrote the above statement before I researched a hypothesis called the "thrifty gene hypothesis" proposed by geneticist James V. Neel in 1962. Neel suggests that evolution (natural selection) whittled down populations favouring those who could get fatter during periods of famine, making fat genes more prevalent. His primary area of interest was diabetes, but the idea was later applied to hypertension and obesity. In the original paper, Neel "envisions diabetes mellitus as an untoward aspect of a 'thriftiness' genotype which is less of an asset now than in the feast-or-famine days of hunting and gathering cultures" (Neel, 1962, p. 360).

The following paragraph which I read on Wikipedia mirrored my own thoughts on the matter almost exactly:

"According to the hypothesis, the 'thrifty' genotype would have been advantageous for hunter-gatherer populations ... because it would allow them to fatten more quickly during times of abundance. Fatter individuals carrying the thrifty genes would thus better survive times of food scarcity. However, *in modern societies with a constant abundance of food, this genotype efficiently prepares individuals for a famine that never comes*. The result of this mismatch between the environment in which the brain evolved and the environment of today is a widespread chronic obesity and related health problems like diabetes" (Wikipedia, 2017, para. 2, my emphasis).

The Palaeolithic Prescription
In 1998, Neel expanded the original hypothesis to a more complex theory of several related diseases such

as type 2 diabetes, obesity, and hypertension caused by the mismatch between our current predicament and our adaption to primitive ecosystems, where people were affected more acutely by environmental changes. As a result, it is suggested that *one possible remedy* (I would suggest the *only* viable remedy) for these conditions is to change both *diet* and *activity* to match our ancestral environment. Neel states: "intervention should be as early as is practical, and consist not just in cutting back on calories while maintaining the standard diet of the high-technology society but incorporating as many elements of the Paleolithic Prescription as possible" (Neel, 1999, p.7).

In his work, Neel was referring to a well-researched book by S. Boyd Eaton et al., entitled *The Paleolithic Prescription* (1988), which suggested that eating and being more active, to mimic the behaviour of our prehistoric ancestors, is the best way to prevent these conditions. Even though it is almost 30 years old, I would recommend this book wholeheartedly, as it is full of excellent arguments and high-quality research as to why we should look to our past to guide our future. It was far ahead of its time, paving the way for many modern hunter-gatherer type diets and exercise programmes. I think that everyone must agree that eating fewer processed foods and becoming more active is a simple, sensible approach to general health and wellbeing. Both Eaton and Neel suggest that eating plenty of natural produce containing protein, good fats and fibre and nutrient-rich carbs combined with adequate exercise is the optimal way to lead a healthy lifestyle.

Prophetic Words

On page 83 of *The Palaeolithic Prescription* (1988), is a section entitled "Shortages", where Eaton et al. state:

"it is likely that they [hunter gatherers or agriculturalists] also faced periodic shortages, great enough to produce weight loss".

This was because food was rarely stored, and when there were shortages, a situation of "perilous deprivation" was created, which may have resulted in death. The authors point out that this problem was solved by natural selection, ie people were "programmed" to gorge during times of plenty, as an insurance policy against times of scarcity. They also state:

"our seemingly insatiable appetites produce fat stores we no longer need. Unless we create a deliberate personal shortage known as dieting, we never used them up".

S. Boyd Eaton and Co. observed, almost 30 years ago, that "our survival (as individuals) is now threatened by plenty instead of by dearth" (Eaton et al., 1988, p. 83)

It is a poor reflection on us as a society that this observation was not taken more seriously back then. Perhaps if it had been, we would not be in the situation we are now, where obesity is now a bigger health issue globally than starvation.

Society cannot be held fully to blame, however. A recent study by researchers at the University of California, San Francisco have made allegations of deception by the sugar industry. This was published in *JAMA Internal Medicine*, has been cited by various news sources, including the *New York Times*. The following extract notes:

"our findings suggest the industry sponsored a research program in the 1960s and 1970s that successfully cast doubt about the hazards of sucrose while promoting fat as the dietary culprit in CHD" (Kearns et al., 2016, abstract)

An article by the *New York Times*, entitled "How The Sugar Industry Shifted Blame To Fat" (O'Connor, 2016), details the seriousness of this and the repercussions that occurred as a result. Dr Stanton Glantz, a professor of medicine at USCF (The Center for Tobacco Control Research and Education), and one of the paper's authors, was quoted in the article as saying: "They were able to derail the discussion about sugar for decades … After the review was published, the debate about sugar and heart disease died down, while low-fat diets gained the endorsement of many health authorities" (O'Connor, 2016, para. 3).

It is very difficult for society to move forward under circumstances where it seems even expert opinion cannot be fully trusted.

Origin of *The Paleolithic Prescription*

The origins of *The Palaeolithic Prescription* can be traced back earlier than Eaton's time, to a book entitled *The Stoneage Diet*, written in 1975 by Walter L. Voegtlin. His idea was based around ecology, ie man as an animal living in a natural environment, and the fact that we were almost exclusively meat-eaters up until about 10,000 years ago. His argument in Chapter 2 ("Low Carbohydrate – An Old 'New Departure' Diet") is that high protein and fat, combined with moderate-to low-carb diets, have been proven to work. He cites examples of their success over a 100-year period (Voegtlin, 1975, pp. 7–13).

Nowadays, there's plenty of solid evidence to further back up Voegtlin's observations, with an array of studies showing that low-carb diets are far more beneficial for weight loss and heart health over low-fat diets. An article by Kris Gunnars, detailing 23 randomized controlled trials, the gold standard of science, can be viewed on the Authority Nutrition's website (Gunnars, 2013).

Some key observations from this article include:

- Low-carb groups often lost two to three times as much weight as the low-fat counterparts.
- In the majority of studies, calories were restricted in the low-fat groups, whereas low-carb groups could generally eat their fill.
- Low-carb diets have a clear advantage when it comes to reducing belly fat.

Whether the thrifty genotype hypothesis is proven true or not, the logic to me seems sound, and is consistent with my journey from obesity to a healthy body weight. However, I think that the feast/famine cycle is even more acute and repetitive than previously suggested. I believe it to be a yearly occurrence, which is triggered by particular food types and because of our symbiotic annual relationship with nature, ie *it intentionally fattens us up through Autumnal produce in order to protect us from the immediate Winter ahead*; and I propose that it is the constant availability of autumnal foods nowadays, ie starchy and sugary carbs, in combination with unhealthy fats, that is the primary cause of chronic weight gain and related health issues.

Thus, it is the moderation of autumnal foods (in particular their refined derivatives), simulating what nature once did for us, that seems to result in fantastic weight loss and health improvements for many individuals, including myself.

Ultimately, this is what the "Don't Eat for Winter" way of eating is all about. Mother Nature used to be our moderator, but now that we have taken her out of the picture and flown the coup, so to speak, we must take personal responsibility and start acting like grownups.

This echoes Voegtlin's dedication at the end of his introduction, where he despairingly dedicates his book to:

"the occasional man, woman, or child who still can resist the specious authority of food merchants, their lavish advertisements and spectacular television commercials and retain sufficient intellectual independence to think for themselves" (Voegtlin, 1975, p. xvii).

I have faith in society and our future because we live in a very different world today. We've woken up as a society thanks to the internet and social media, which have helped disseminate independent knowledge faster than ever before. We've also become aware of the recent revelations regarding how the sugar industry influenced top scientific research a half century ago, in order to convince the world that low-fat/high-carb diets were the healthiest choice. However, this has been proven incorrect through the stark statistics regarding the rising levels of illness and death caused by obesity, which has overtaken malnutrition across the globe. We have no choice but to wake up, and if we don't, things will continue to worsen.

Introduction to The DEFoW Diet

Don't Eat For Winter, or The DEFoW Diet for short, is a type of Palaeolithic Prescription, or a set of guidelines, for those who are overweight and want to trim down to their ideal shape, in order to become the summer, hunter version of themselves. It focuses on eating mainly staple foods that are available throughout the year, with plenty of fibrous spring/summer, low GI (Glycemic Index) foods. It also recommends carefully considering the amount of autumnal starchy and sugary foods (ie carbs) eaten, particularly in conjunction with fats, in order to avoid the natural combinations that trigger instinctual binge eating. This method will allow us to curtail the body's natural fat storage process. Of course, regular exercise is also recommended, but there's no point in killing yourself in the gym or pounding the road without a sensible diet to support your activities, in order to recover well and to maximise the results of your efforts.

These triggers are powerful and are programmed into us to encourage the storage of future energy in the form of fat. This is for our own protection and survival because, when the world was wild and food was scarce, you had to put on weight when you had the opportunity before winter, or you wouldn't survive for very long.

Foods designed to trigger these responses are now readily available (almost) everywhere because of human ingenuity. However, we have not yet evolved and adapted enough biologically in order to cope with this abundance. Do we want to adapt to an artificial environment anyway? If we adapt to an artificial environment, what happens if that ever fails? To counter this problem, we need to be just as clever about how we eat, in order to avoid chronic overstimulation of the protection mechanisms that nature has given us.

I'll rephrase this, because it's important:

Now that we've *used our intelligence to overcome nature*, and autumnal foods are available 24/7/365, in both their natural and processed/refined forms, *we need to use that same intelligence, in* an equal but opposite manner, to overcome our natural instinct to overeat, in order to avoid becoming obese.

One more time, put in yet another way because it is *really, really* important:

Our survival instincts motivated us to create an over-abundance of food *in order to prevent death* caused by starvation. *Ironically, the solution has caused more death* in the form of chronic obesity and related health issues, because we have not learned to control our instincts to overconsume.

This is really quite stark and almost grotesque. The survival instincts that drove us to solve death have led to more death. Solving one problem has caused another. Preventing starvation has led to chronic obesity, the definitive flip-flop, and now overeating is quickly becoming an even bigger cause of death than malnutrition.

The fact that a gift from nature, ie the ability to store energy (as fat), in order to survive, is now the cause of major health issues across the planet, shows how far we've separated ourselves from nature. But, it's not too late: we can come back from this through understanding that we are part of nature and need to work with it and not against it, as we have defiantly done. This is at the core of The DEFoW Diet.

The method of achieving this with The DEFoW Diet is through *moderating the consumption of autumnal produce* in particular, which, as discussed, is designed by nature to fatten us up for the winter. These foods would simply not be available to us all year around were we living closer to the natural environment in which we evolved, so we need to take responsibility and moderate them, just as nature once did for us.

So, it's simple really: "Don't Eat for Winter", at least not all of the time, unless you want to gain weight!

Note: If you are wondering at this point what a carb is, and what autumnal foods are, don't worry, we will get into the nitty gritty all of that soon. Essentially, think of anything typically harvested in autumn, for example fruits, crops, potatoes, root veg etc. All of these foods contain either starch or sugars (this is plant energy or plant fat, and a lot of sunlight is needed to create it, which is why they are harvested at the end of summer). Starch is simply a pre-digested form of sugar and is readily converted into sugar once in your stomach. In essence, autumnal foods are predominantly foods rich in sugar or starch, ie carbs. What makes things worse is that they taste so good, because nature programmed us to eat lots of them when they become available, and by refining the sugars from these foods we can create marvellous-tasting goodies from candies to cakes.

Don't say the "D" word

The word *diet* has negative connotations. When someone thinks about the word diet, they tend to think about calorie restriction, denial, misery, hunger, punishment, guilt, starvation and cravings, among other things. There is a huge difference, however, between the terms "going on a diet" and eating a "sensible diet".

Some people go on fad diets, and eat lots of low-calorie items like cabbage soup and salads for a month, or follow a plan where they have to count up calories in everything they eat (perhaps in a simplified form), in order to create a calorie deficit. Others include meal replacements, which essentially help to enforce a calorie deficit too. These sorts of diets may not be healthy for either mind and body over prolonged periods of time, because they are essentially a form of self-denial, which typically we rebel against. It's like mistreating a dog for too long: at some point the dog will get vicious and bite back. I'm all for a little bit of short-term fasting here and there, and there are real health benefits to it as it helps clear out junk from our cells. The discoveries by Nobel Prize winner Yoshinori Ohsumi, on the mechanisms of autophagy, highlight this. However, a long-term calorie-restricted diet with low amounts of fats, carbs and proteins means your body may lose more than just fat over the course of the diet. It may also lose muscle, and may struggle to function correctly, as these nutrients are crucial to hormone function, energy levels and repair.

Once an individual gets to the end of the diet, their body is crying out for calories and nutrients, and, as a result, often powerful binge-eating instincts float to the surface. Your body is a biological machine designed for survival: when it is deprived, it will switch into a different mode to protect brain and body; and your metabolism slows down to prolong your survival by slowing down the rate at which it burns energy. As soon as normal eating resumes, it will feast on whatever is at hand in a frenzy, because it assumes another famine is around the corner; and the fact that your metabolism has slowed down compounds the problem, as you then gain weight at an accelerated rate because you're not burning energy as quickly as you were before you deprived yourself.

The term diet, in the case of The DEFoW Diet, simply means some sensible daily choices and some basic guidelines that ensure you get enough fat, protein, fibre, vitamins, minerals, *and* the precise amount of carbs to keep you full of energy and in tip-top shape. At its most basic, if focuses, in particular, on more controlled carb intake based on your daily energy requirements, which you will more fully understand by the end of the book.

There are three main nutrients (macronutrients) that the body needs – fats, proteins and carbs. Put in simple terms, fat is used for body function, particularly hormones, and also as a slow burning, efficient, energy source; protein builds and repairs muscle; and carbs give you instant fast burning energy, primarily for brain function and intense physical activity. Fibre is often present with carbs (for example the skin of an apple, the bran or shell of wholegrains etc), contains vitamins and minerals, and assists with passing food through the bowel. It also slows down the process of digesting the food and thus assists with a slower, more constant supply of sugar to the blood stream, providing this form of energy over a longer period.

As well as macronutrients, there are micronutrients (vitamins and minerals), such as vitamin D3, which helps us absorb calcium, a mineral, which is one of the building blocks of bones and teeth, as well as being an important electrolyte.

If you provide your body with an ample supply of these nutrients, in conjunction with water, sunlight and decent air, you will thrive, just like a plant thrives when you give it the right fertilizer along with the correct amount of water and adequate sunlight. A thriving plant in flower looks spectacular and is more resistant to disease. Just like a plant, if you give your body all that it requires, your body will automatically create the best version of itself, given enough time, and you will begin to look and feel amazing.

With all this in mind, The DEFoW Diet gives you the tools to make the right choices. It's not about big fancy recipes, or depriving yourself of calories – it's about explaining what you need to eat, when you need to eat it, and most importantly why – in order keep your motor humming and to transform you into the best version of yourself. Once you know these things, you will still have choices to make because the world is full temptations. Of course, you can still have treats, and you should not feel any guilt when eating them. But, equally, you will be armed with the knowledge of what happens to your body when you indulge on them. If you make the right choices most of the time (80/20 rule), you'll see terrific results. I certainly did.

Knowledge + Action = Power!

Chapter 2

My Story

(The closet athlete)

You can't out-train ignorance

My Story

The Closet Athlete

My name is Cian Foley. I hail from a city in Ireland called Waterford. I want to tell you about my journey from an 18-stone (115-kilogram) couch potato to a 12-stone (<78-kilogram) Irish, European and World Kettlebell Champion in the space of a few short years. The transition would have been much faster and easier had I known then what I know now; but I had to do it the hard way and discover what worked for me bit by bit, as I was totally ignorant of diet in the beginning. However, it won't be as tough or take as long for you, if you take the time to absorb the information contained in this book.

My story is not unique. I was an overweight kid: my nickname in school was "Chubby" (kids can be so cruel). If I had been a sensitive kid, I would have found that very hurtful, but I was oblivious to it until I was a teenager, when I became self-conscious enough for it to bother me. It obviously affected me a lot, because during my teens I dieted excessively, which had my father worried. One day, he gave out to me angrily saying: "You're gone too skinny!" His anger that day gave me a sense of defiant achievement, which, on reflection, showed that I had some sort of underlying

41

esteem issues. I used to have to starve myself to be slim.

During that time, I got to a good level of fitness and managed to knock off all of my childhood puppy fat. I showed promise as a cyclist and martial artist, and reached a solid level at both sports, using weight training to assist with both.

Gain and Pain

After I finished school, I went to college to study computer science and, once I graduated, I got a desk job in my local university as a software developer/researcher. I got married to my lovely wife, Nicola, and soon after we had two beautiful children, Sian and Daniel. Over the course of 10 years, I let myself go and put on about 80+ pounds of fat or six stone, just shy of 40 kilograms.

Back then, I ate pizzas, burgers, fries with taco meat loaded with cheese, drank gallons of fizzy drinks, ate sweets and treats without moderation, and had all the habits you'd expect an overweight person to have. How my body survived this is a testament to the resilience of our most valuable asset.

By my early 30s, I was getting pains in my chest, groin, feet and knees, and my skin wasn't great. I looked puffy and swollen, felt bad a lot of the time and I really thought my life was practically over.

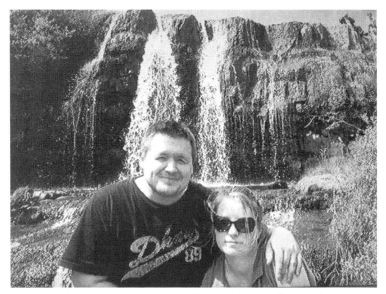

The overweight version of me, with my wife, Nicola

I was playing a bit of squash at this point too and this helped me fool myself into believing that I was doing my best to get fit; but there was no way I could ever out-train my own ignorance, and the extra weight was actually causing joint pains. I was uneducated, and when I look back I feel sorry for that guy: he tried hard, but was caught in the Matrix and, I can assure you, ignorance was not bliss.

The Road to ~~Damascus~~ Waterford

The real change began in 2011. I decided to try to get fit and lose enough weight to take on the Inca Trail in

43

Peru, with my wife Nicola, for the Irish Red Cross charity. So, I began walking the local mountains in order to get fit. This helped me to lose about a stone (five to six kilograms) over a six-month period, enough to ensure that I completed the trek and became a much fitter, happier, healthier person. At this point, I thought that I was in decent shape. When I look back at the photographs, I realise that I was only getting started. I was fitter, but still very overweight.

After Machu Picchu, I kept up the hiking and being active. Soon after, I took on another challenge – a kind of triathlon with a difference, with a good friend of mine, Kieran O'Sullivan. We cycled 20 miles, hiked up to and swam a local corrie lake in the mountains, and then hiked back down and cycled home to Waterford. We were both very tired after it, but Kieran was impressed with how I dealt with the challenge. During the cycle, Kieran said a few words to me that sent me into a chain reaction of positivity. He said: "You're a closet athlete!" These words resonated with me and I started to believe in myself.

Before that day, I felt my life was pretty much over from a sporting point of view. I was very wrong, and underestimated the resilience of the human body. I also underestimated the power of positivity. So, if you see someone else trying their best and achieving, encourage them and be excited for them; and if someone encourages you, absorb the compliment and accept it with open arms.

After that day, Kieran encouraged me to take part in a circuit training class he went to. I did my first circuit with him and suffered DOMS (delayed onset muscle soreness) for about two weeks because, I used muscles I hadn't exercised in about 10 years. The instructor told me later he thought I'd never be back, but I did go back and did another class and I was sore again for another week. After some time, I did a second class a week and a third and stuck at it and started to enjoy it. So, don't give up if you feel really sore after your first session of exercise. It's normal, but it gets easier.

Setting Goals

This went on for about six months, and at the end of 2012, I took part in my first kettlebell sport (Girevoy Sport or GS) competition, which was the tool of choice at the gym. A kettlebell is a metal ball with a handle and a very versatile piece of exercise equipment. Kettlebell sport is about lifting a kettlebell for as many repetitions as possible in a set time (normally 10 minutes). I weighed in at 99 kilograms (15 stone 8 pounds) and competed with a pair of 16-kilogram kettlebells in a five-minute competition.

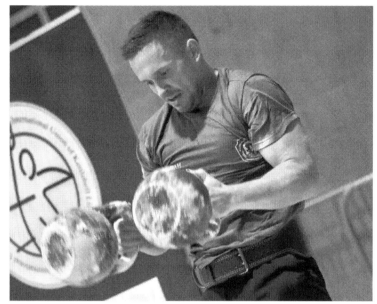

Competing at the IUKL Kettlebell Sport World Championships,
Dublin, Ireland 2015
(Photo Credit: Anton Krieger)

To my surprise, I won my category, so I was beginning to get relatively fit, but I still wasn't in shape. At this point I created a goal in my head: I wanted to get into lower-weight categories in kettlebell sport to compete against people with the same lean body mass as myself. The lighter I could get, the more competitive I would be in that category. My goal for weight loss wasn't vanity, it was for sport, and I was on a mission.

You Can't Out-train Ignorance

It was then that I first heard the phrase, "You can't out-train a bad diet." The truth was, I was in denial and thought I could work off my body fat through punishing myself at the gym, but it simply wasn't possible with the types of food I was eating, and the way I was eating them. I didn't even really know what a bad diet was, so how could I fix that problem in my state of ignorance? Far too often I see people who are training away in a similar state of ignorance, which is very disheartening for them, because after months and months of dedication and training, they see very little physical change. It doesn't need to be this difficult. This will *not* be the case with you.

Slowly, I came to the realisation that I had to look more closely at my diet and tried a few different diets, to really cut my weight. It was then that I began eating more natural foods and cut down on starchy carbs and refined sugars, eating more protein and fats. I went from 15 stone eight pounds (99 kilograms) to 13 stone eight pounds (86 kilograms), a six-month loss of almost two stone. I was getting complimented every time I met anyone who knew me, and that felt fantastic and wanted more and more of the same. Now I had two reasons to cut weight: (a) for kettlebell sport competitions and (b) to get positive feedback on my appearance. I know this sounds a bit ego-driven, but because I'd spent 10 years feeling disgusted with myself, it was an amazing feeling to receive compliments on my physical appearance. I still find it difficult to rationalise, but it feels great, I won't lie to you; and I don't think anyone could ever get fed up with that.

The amazing thing about all of this weight loss is that I can say, hand on heart, that I was never hungry. What confused me was that much of the food was very calorie dense (lots of fats for example), yet I lost weight. Then I started researching the why ...

Applying a Computer Science Background

My professional background is in Research and Software Engineering, and I experimented on my body for sporting purposes as if it were a piece of hardware with controlling software. I am fluent with logic and systems that take input variables and produce different outputs depending on these parameters. Therefore, I see the body as something very similar to a programmable machine, albeit an amazingly complex one. However, there are some fundamental input variables, which, if tweaked correctly, result in incredible changes over time. I've read books and papers, scoured the internet, spoken to dieticians, medical doctors, health specialists and other athletes about these inputs, and, most importantly, applied the knowledge to my own body for weight control and energy production. What stood out was that tweaking carbs lead to increased energy and fat loss, and it bothered me as to why this was the case, when I'd been brought up with the notion that low-fat diets were the way to go for losing fat. After much contemplation, I had the definitive "Eureka" moment, and came up with the Don't Eat for Winter concept, ie:

Perpetually eating Autumnal foods and derivatives without moderation leads to chronic weight gain to prepare your body for a winter that never comes, and therefore doing the opposite should lead to weight loss.

This is a simple, common sense hypothesis, which I've backed up with data and research in this book. Perhaps things will change for the better when we begin to moderate autumnal foods correctly. As stated previously, before modern intervention, Mother Nature was that moderator and gave us the optimal foods for our needs for the seasons that lay immediately ahead; but now that we've taken her out of the equation, we've got to be more responsible and undertake that moderation ourselves.

One final point on this is related to change. A quote used by Alcoholics Anonymous, often attributed to Albert Einstein, sums it up nicely: "The definition of insanity is doing something over and over again and expecting a different result." We have repeated and propagated a mistake over and over, and the world is very sick. How could we have gone so far wrong? We need to change something, or nothing will ever change. I discovered that change for myself over the course of many years of trial and error and the results are flabbergasting. Hopefully, it will be a catalyst for change in others, too. No more trial and error: trial and success from now on!

Getting it Right for You

Everyone is different to some extent, and so foods affect us to varying degrees. Yet, we are all fundamentally the same, ie we use food for energy and maintenance of our bodies and excess energy is stored as fat. Human breast milk is practically identical in terms of nutrient ratios the world over, so human babies across the world are generally fed in exactly the same way. The inputs are the same. If we were that different, baby milk wouldn't be a one-size-fits-all formula. I'm not coming up with any new science here: I'm simply putting forward a fundamental reason for why this type of eating has worked so well for me. For some time, I understood *how* I lost the weight, *but I only recently discovered the why.*

After getting the diet right, I became both fit and in shape and it became evident that it was working in 2015, when I became an IUKL European (Varna, Bulgaria) and World Champion (Dublin, Ireland) in

Kettlebell lifting in the adult men's <85-kilogram body weight category, using 2 x 24-kilogram kettlebells, in a very competitive division.

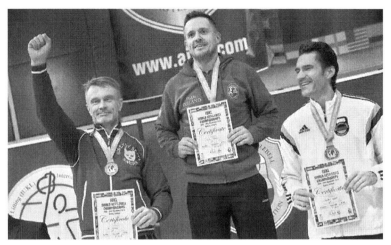

Winning Gold for Ireland at the IUKL Kettlebell World Championship
Amateur Mens Long Cycle <85kg, Dublin, Ireland 2016
Left to Right: Per Olhans, Cian Foley, Karsten Bollert
(Photo Credit: Anton Krieger)

I was honoured to place first in a field of 14 other competitors from across the world – champions in their own countries – and I am very grateful to my coach, Rosaleen Flynn, for the training programme she laid out for me for this competition.

However, this was still not the end of my transformation: I was applying the rules of the diet to a large degree, but still didn't fully understand the why. Once I figured out the why, the how became so much simpler, and within eight weeks, through following the

Don't Eat for Winter (DEFoW diet) myself, I lost a final 8 kilograms that I was holding on to, settling at about 77 kilograms, revealing abs and muscles I didn't even know I had.

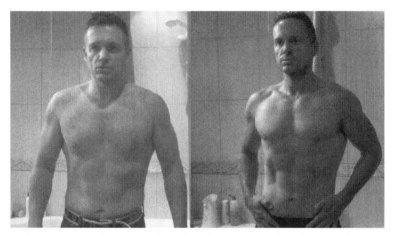

My final transformation (age 40) after I stopped eating for winter

I did this completely naturally, without ever feeling hungry or counting calories and, most importantly, without drugs. This allowed me to then water cut (ie draining as much water from the body as possible for a competition, which I don't recommend) to a weight of 72.85 kilograms (a total loss of 42 kilograms, more than half of my current body weight) and competed in the European Kettlebell Championships (in Poland, May 2016) in the <73-kilogram body weight category, two full weight categories lower than the one I competed in 2015, when I won the European and World Championships.

I've maintained my weight at <80 kilograms for about a year now, without any hardship at all. I've demonstrated that I can now maintain my weight without difficulty, in the full confidence that I will never again become obese (once I continue to stick to the basic principles of the diet).

In summary, I thought my life was over at 35, getting pains everywhere – chest, groin, knees, feet – and just feeling bad all the time. I never thought my life would change so drastically. It didn't happen quickly for me, due to a lack of knowledge, and I had to make adjustments to my diet as I discovered each subsequent step. This eventually resulted in the eureka moment of the 'Don't Eat for Winter' concept; a new, simple way of thinking about food, and a method of eating (The DEFoW Diet) that has changed everything for me, and I am privileged to share it with you.

With this knowledge, I am certain that your transformation will be far quicker than mine and should you wish to share your success story with me and others, to inspire us, please do so here:

www.donteatforwinter.com/testimonials

Chapter 3

There's *NO* Starch in March

(or February or April or May or …)

Nature provides us with the ideal foods in autumn to trigger weight gain, in order to help us survive the oncoming winter

There's *NO* Starch in March

GI Whizz!!! Why Did We Not Spot This???

Before modern farming and storage, there were only a few staples constantly available all year around, such as meat, fish, poultry and eggs. Plant produce was seasonal and so only formed part of the diet, as and when it became available. Most of the staples, and indeed vegetation for most of the year (besides autumn), have zero or low position on the Glycemic Index, or a low GI.

The GI is an index of various foods and their effect on blood sugar levels, rated on a scale of 0 to 100 (and beyond), where 100 is the response of the body to glucose.

In spring and early summer, the berries and veg available, in general, have a low GI. In late summer and autumn (and even into winter), however, many sweet fruits, tubers, cereals and root veg appear, and these typically have a mid to high GI. Jacket potatoes and white rice, and even root veg, like carrots and parsnips, are very high on the GI and when eaten, cause sugar to enter the blood stream quickly. This in turn results in an insulin response, which we will discuss later.

In order to back up my Don't Eat for Winter hypothesis, I constructed a spreadsheet with most of the indigenous fruit and veg available in the UK and Ireland, and organised them into their natural harvesting months. I then researched each food's GI value from University of Sydney's GI database, Harvard's GI tables of common foods, and other resources, and stored that data with the food item in a spreadsheet. I then totalled and averaged the data and graphed it (for further details, please visit www.donteatforwinter.com/theory).

What I found supported my common-sense hypothesis in a startling way: that nature provided us with the ideal foods in autumn (ie starch and sugar), to promote immediate weight gain, in order to survive the winter.

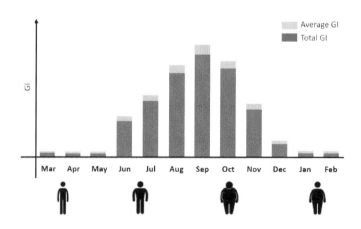

Figure 1 – Total & Average GI of Natural Monthly Produce

The graph above shows the total GI of foods available during each month in blue, with the average in red. It is very effective in illustrating that nature produces more foods with a higher GI during late summer and autumn, peaking in September.

The conclusion that I would suggest from these findings is that the spike in carb-rich produce, ie sugary and starchy, high GI foods, available in autumn, prepared human beings for winter by triggering processes in the body that encourage fat storage, so that they could survive a subsequent period with less available food and with colder weather, ie winter and early spring. The stickmen beneath the graph bars give a simplified and exaggerated depiction of the weight gain and loss cycle over a 12-month period.

In my opinion, and in my experience, eating these sorts of foods in either their natural or processed form, every day, and without moderation, leads to perpetual weight gain for a multitude of reasons, which we will delve into later. Ultimately, they are designed by nature to make humans (and animals) as fat as possible, in as short a time as possible, in order to protect and keep them alive. Nature has seduced us, giving us a sweet tooth, and cravings for carbs, in order to encourage us to eat more of this type of food, especially in conjunction with fats, which, as well as being present in the staples, also become abundant at this time of year in the form of nuts. Some of these combinations include fruit and nuts, bread and butter, pies, tarts, cakes, battered fish, pizzas, chocolate, etc. This is all the stuff that tastes really nice, which is no coincidence, either.

How Fat Can a Human Get before Winter?

Fat is essentially a backup battery for human beings. It is stored on our bodies when we overeat and converted back into energy that can be used during low-level aerobic activity, for example walking, breathing and resting. If you breathe and your heart beats, your body will automatically burn fat once your blood sugar levels are normal.

Fat is an extremely efficient form of energy storage. According to many sources, including the Mayo Clinic (2017, para. 7), there are about 3,500 calories in a pound (0.45 kilograms) of body fat, which equates to about 7,700 calories per kilogram. This would give an average resting human being enough energy for approximately two days per pound, or four days per kilogram of body fat.

In order to gain 1lb of fat, a person would need to consume a surplus of 3,500 calories over their normal energy requirements. Over a single day, this sort of excess would be practically impossible to achieve, but over the course of a week, it would be possible. It can therefore be deduced that eating a *surplus* of 500 calories a day for three months would yield gains of about 14 pounds, one stone or six kilograms (there are many variables here and I am only speaking in very approximate terms). This is a significant amount of energy stored and would certainly help a human to survive the food shortages that follow in winter and early spring.

A surplus of calories would not be difficult to achieve in autumn, with the availability of energy-dense foods such as sweet fruits, starchy grains and root veg along with fatty foods like nuts and of course the fatty and oily staples such as meat, fish and eggs, which are available all year round. Eating a couple of apples, with a handful of hazelnuts (say 50g), would provide the body with over 500 calories. This is based on Google Search Engine's conversion tool, which uses the USDA Food Composition Database as one of its sources http://ndb.nal.usda.gov – a fantastic database for discovering the macro and micronutrient content of foods. This could easily be collected and consumed, along with a person's regular diet, every day during late summer and autumn, creating a surplus and facilitating significant weight gain over the course of only a few short months.

Of course, as food became scarce again, that surplus would flip to a deficit during the worst parts of winter and early spring, and the weight gained will simply be used as energy, and fall away naturally, as intended. It was only gained because of evolutionary processes which helped humans, and other creatures, to use the tools available to survive a recurring period of famine and cold. The weight gained would not have been significant enough, or stay deposited on the body long enough to cause any health issues, unlike the perpetual weight gain facilitated by the modern era of supermarkets and fast food chains, filled with autumnal produce, all year long, and in particular their plethora of processed derivatives.

The arguments above are presented based solely on calorie excess alone. I believe there is more to it than that however, and the reasons for weight gain are multifactorial, including:

1. **Calorie surplus, and less energy expenditure, because of abundance:** in particular, specific types of carbs, which only exist in parts of the world with pronounced seasons for short periods. Other parts of the world have different seasons with their own feast and famine cycles, such as the tropical wet/dry (summer/winter) seasons of the equator.

2. **The response of our bodies to excess carb or sugar energy:** and the resulting insulin response, which

causes the body's cells to go into storage mode, which we will deal with in due course.

3. **The effects that carbs, amplified with the presence of fats, have on our brains**: encouraging us to binge eat and want to eat more (try eating just one square of chocolate!).

In essence, we are designed to store energy in the form of fat quickly, and use it slowly. It is typically easier to gain weight than it is to lose it, as we all know. Putting up weight is natural and healthy, once it does not become chronic and perpetual, so we need to consider that our eating habits are now out of sync with nature and the way it has cleverly adapted and shaped our bodies and minds over countless millennia. We need to restore our natural eating habits as best as possible, in order to become the optimum version of ourselves.

What does Eating for Winter Mean?

Eating for winter simply means eating autumnal foods (and processed derivatives) with every meal, without consideration or any form of moderation. Autumnal foods include cereal crops, potatoes, rice, fruits, starchy veg, and all processed derivatives of same, such as breads, cakes, chips, fries, rice products, pastas, refined sugars, fruit juices, dried fruits, breakfast cereals and so on – basically comfort food. This is the stuff that tastes really good, and on which we typically find ourselves grazing over the course of the day. The processed versions of these foods are often combined with fats to make them even tastier. I term this "The Squirrel Formula".

The Squirrel Formula – Not Totally Nuts!

It is the types of food available, and not the approaching cold in autumn that sends squirrels into a frenzy of eating and storing food for the impending winter. Last year (2016), because of the warm winter, there was an obesity epidemic among the squirrel population (Jamieson, 2016). This highlights the fact that a squirrel does not consciously know winter is coming and suddenly decides to start eating and storing food. Rather, something naturally triggers its instincts to eat and put on weight and keep eating and putting on weight while this type of food is available (like us and supermarkets). Nature triggers this eating through the types of food available to the squirrel at this time of year. Is it simply because of abundance, or other factors?

We are very similar to squirrels, in that we are excellent gatherers. Food, however, is perishable, and in our past, nature did the thinking for us and supplied us with different types of foods at different times of the year. Though we could store things like nuts for some time, in general we ate what nature gave us, as it became available. We adapted to these conditions and what we are today is a result of this adaptation. Fortunately (and unfortunately), due to our ingenuity, we have become the ultimate gatherers and have learnt how to store and preserve practically everything, so it can be eaten at any time of the year. This started with processes such as salting meat, storing fish in ice houses, and storing grain in granaries, but developed, over the years, into adding preservatives, deep freezer storage, vacuum packing, genetic engineering etc. This ingenuity must be matched now in an equal but opposite measure, and we must use our grey matter to out-think our instincts and moderate our consumption of these autumnal foods and derivatives, in order to overcome the natural triggers that lead to binge eating. If we don't, we will suffer the same fate indefinitely, and the chronic obesity epidemic, which is already catastrophic, will continue to worsen.

Hi(GI)bernation

Another example of this trigger is seen in hibernating animals that eat fruits, nuts and their staples, in order to get really fat over the autumn. They instinctually put on this weight, which allows them to survive through the winter by slowly burning off excess body fat while sleeping, and provides them with enough energy to survive for months. These creatures have evolved to a point where they do not even bother staying awake during the winter, as there is so little food available in their environment, and conditions are so harsh. They happily live off the body fat they accumulated during the autumn.

We are part of the same animal kingdom, so similar rules apply to us, and although we don't hibernate, the high availability of high GI carbohydrates does affect us, and causes us to get fat.

Instinctual Calorie Bomb

It has been shown the high GI of carbs affects our brains in similar ways to drugs. According to a study entitled "Effects of Dietary Glycemic Index on Brain Regions Related to Reward and Craving in Men", published by the *American Journal of Clinical Nutrition*, Lennerz et al. concluded: "Compared with an isocaloric low GI meal, a high GI meal decreased plasma glucose, increased hunger, and selectively stimulated brain regions associated with reward and craving in the late postprandial period" (Lennerz et al., 2013, p. 1).

In an article posted on the Harvard Medical School website, David Ludwig, HMS Professor of Pediatrics at Boston Children's Hospital, and team lead of the study, said: "These findings suggest that limiting high-glycemic index carbs like white bread and potatoes could help obese individuals reduce cravings and control the urge to overeat" (Mooney, 2013, para. 9).

You've often heard of food tasting of "more". You cannot stop eating something because it tastes so good. We no longer listen to reason and make up excuses on why the proverbial "one more" is no harm. Then afterwards we feel low because we are disappointed that our will power wasn't powerful enough to overcome these urges.

This is an example of our subconscious instincts overriding our conscious thoughts for a particular reason. I would suggest that the reason is the continuation of our species, or, in other words, survival. If we were not programmed this way, we would have died off as a species well before now. The reason these foods taste so nice is because they trigger our primal instincts. I, for one, suffer terribly from this. Once I start eating foods of this type, I become an insatiable creature, searching the cupboards of my house for treats, etc, and I have felt terrible afterwards because at the time I could not overcome these urges with willpower alone. I have felt shame, disappointment, self-loathing, etc, because I believe that I've ruined all my hard work training in the gym or being good all day. Of course, I realise now that it was never my fault – nature made me this way in order that I might survive a much harsher period that my ancestors had to endure, and this is part of my heritage. Modern society has strayed far from this environment, but my genes have not.

Take Back the Power

From now on, you should not feel guilty about your instincts, but you should become acutely aware of them and how much power they can have over you.

The first step is awareness, because once you are aware, you can prevent them from overpowering your will by simply avoiding the triggers that set off the bomb. Prevention is always better than cure.

It is ironic that these instincts, which were designed to protect us, are now killing us through obesity-related health problems. We are being destroyed by our own ingenuity, like some sort of strange curse. That is why it is so important for us to understand this, applying the same intelligence we used to create this problem to solve it – to start eating more like our ancestors, who were moderated by nature, a harsh but fair mother. For them, high GI foods were much less available for nine months of the year, so they didn't have the option of getting into the eating frenzies that many of us go through daily.

Unfortunately, these days, avoiding the types of foods that set off your instincts is almost impossible. Walking into a convenience store is like running the gauntlet.

These foods are everywhere, packaged up beautifully and in your face, and it is very difficult to walk out without a tasty treat containing these instinct-inducing foods. Be warned, though, if you do eat one, it will set off the bomb in your brain and you will not be satisfied. You will want more, just like the squirrels do; and, unless you are extremely disciplined and iron-willed, you will succumb. So, the simplest thing is not to start in the first place.

Processed foods and all commercial goods are designed to sell and make money for a business. Manufacturers create things that taste nice and prey on these instincts, which subconsciously force you to buy them. It's not magic: it's nature. The reason they taste nice is because our bodies recognise them as foods that will make us gain weight, in order to survive. There must be some natural reason for them to taste so good to us; after all, taste is subjective and molecules are just combinations of atoms. It's only because we evolved symbiotically with nature that certain foods taste really good to us, on account of their benefit to us. Back then, getting fat quick to prepare for the famine of winter was a very important skill to have, and so instinctively recognising the foods that achieve this goal was critical. The net effect is that that these foods taste incredible but yet do satiate us, we simply want more and more.

It's nobody's fault that this is the case: it just is, and business is business, especially when not fully regulated; and how could it be regulated, when all the facts are still not fully understood? These products sell because they satisfy our instincts and give us instant gratification, but the feel-good-factor is short-lived and soon, we begin to crave more.

I have heard it suggested that there is some sort of conspiracy to make us all fat and unhealthy, so that we end up dependent on pharmaceuticals. I don't buy this at all, and think it is much simpler than this. It's down to commerce. Businesses has discovered a natural formula that appeals to our survival instincts through trial and error – a combination of refined sugars and fats in particular. They make things that taste incredible, because things that taste incredible sell, and though it may not be moral to prey on instincts, either consciously or innocently, it makes good business sense to produce things that people will purchase on impulse. Unfortunately for us, without knowledge, we will just keep buying and buying them because they make us feel good while we eat them; but it's just a quick hit, and over time they will make us feel bad, gain weight and eventually, become unhealthy.

Natural combinations of foods can also cause these triggers and even though they can be quite healthy for us, they may cause weight gain too – for example, a peanut butter and jam (jelly) sandwich, or trail mixes with nuts and dried fruit. Unfortunately, these foods cause the same instinct invocation and should be eaten in moderation. If you just ate the nuts alone, you would be more satiated and less likely to deposit fat. All of this will be explored as we go on.

In summary, eating high GI foods, especially in combination with fats, is what I call Eating for Winter, or "The Squirrel Formula". Our instincts are invoked and set off a chain reaction type bomb in our brains, which pleads with us to eat more and more of it, making all sorts of excuses as to justify it; and more often than not, we obey. This results in our storing the excess energy in an explosion of fat storage – the proverbial calorie bomb. Not only that – we get feelings of guilt and shame afterwards because there is a stigma in modern society about being overweight. None of this is your fault: your design is simply being exploited.

Don't Eat for Winter, or The DEFoW Diet for short, is a way of eating that cleverly avoids triggering our instincts from going into overdrive, by selecting foods that disarm the bomb's detonator.

We Go Ga-Ga for Mother Nature's Milk

To further back up the points made above, about the combinations of autumnal foods and fats triggering instincts, there is one signature food that is designed to make human beings put on as much weight as possible (muscle, fat, bone etc) in as short a space of time as possible, and that is, *human breast milk*. We need only look at the ratio of macronutrients in it to discover why.

Aside: macronutrient ratios are simply the ratios of calories in a diet from nutrients that make up the largest parts of our diet, ie carbs, protein and fat, as opposed to micronutrients like vitamins and minerals, which are necessary but are not needed in very large quantities. These nutrients can be seen itemised on the labelling of most processed products. The micronutrients are often listed too, showing mineral and vitamin content. Natural foods often don't have labels, but a quick search online will tell you exactly the quantities of each macro and micronutrient in a food. A site with an enormous database of foods breakdown can be found here: http://ndb.nal.usda.gov

In human breast milk, the macronutrient ratio is roughly 10% protein, 50% fat and 40% lactose (ie sugar or carbs). This is the ideal formula for depositing mass on a human baby's body, as decided by nature since time began. If nature decided it, it must be optimal.

In the natural world, during the first half of the year there is very little sugar or starch available. Staples include meat, seafood and eggs, and so the macronutrient ratio is very different from baby milk and would be something like a bodybuilder's diet, with high protein and fat, and low carbs. Perhaps 40% protein, 40% fat and 20% carbs. In autumn, however, the macronutrient ratio of food produced by nature goes from a low percentage of carbs *to a high percentage of carbs,* compared to protein and fat. A glut of high GI fruits, veg, cereals and so on becomes available from May through October, as presented in Figure 1. In other words, in autumn, the macronutrient ratio tends towards the ratios found in human breast milk, as more carbs and nuts become available and easily harvestable. Perhaps 20% protein, 40% fat and 40% carbs.

The Earth seems to become analogous to a source of mother's milk, fattening and hardening up her children in order to increase their chances of surviving winter (and why wouldn't she, as we are part of her ecosystem?). Again, nature does things optimally and so the ratios are designed, through evolution, to be perfect for our survival requirements.

Tip: watch out for similar ratios in everyday foods. The macronutrients are written on the packaging of most processed foods. Avoid high-carb foods, in particular refined sugar based high GI carbs, and especially those containing lots of fat too. It stands to reason that we like to guzzle foods with these types of ratios as our brains are hard wired to want more, just as we did when we were hungry little babies wanting for mommy's milk.

Chapter 4

The Science Bit

(All calories are equal, but some calories are more equal than others)

Proteins, fats and fibrous foods are far more beneficial to our body health than more starchy and sugary high GI foods, which are, in general, primarily utilised for energy

The Science Bit

Insulin(ce)!!!

Surely you're not suggesting carbs actually trigger fat storage?

It is carbs that affect our blood sugar levels more than any other macronutrient and they come in two main forms: starchy foods (for example starchy veg, grains, corn, rice, potatoes, etc) and sugary foods (fructose in fruit, lactose in milk, etc). Food containing a lot of fibre generally lowers the GI of the food, because it slows down the digestion of the sugar/starch (fibre also helps to lower bad cholesterol and clear waste, so eat plenty!), but it does not affect the total amount of sugar energy ingested or the Glycemic Load (GL) and so GL can be a more important measure from that perspective. The GI and GL of food is very important for diabetics to understand, as they must take great care to manage their blood sugar levels.

Tip: you can search for a food's GI at The University of Sydney's website: www.glycemicindex.com. In general, if something is sweet or starchy it has a high GI and includes many unexpected foods at the high end of the scale, including veg like parsnips and turnips.

Fat Storage Mode

When you eat carbs, your stomach will process them and glucose will enter your blood stream. Insulin hormone is produced by the pancreas in response to deal with the invasion of glucose, so that the energy can be managed, ie used/stored effectively. Glucose gets converted to glycogen and is stored in your muscles and liver for short-term energy usage. The excess is converted into fat and stored in fat cells for future energy use.

When your body produces insulin, it signals to your cells to receive protein, fat and sugar. Your body will also produce insulin when you eat protein, but it is far less pronounced in comparison to eating carbs, especially large quantities of high GI carbs, which are common in many convenience foods.

According to an article on HowStuffWorks, by author Craig Freudenrich, PhD, it takes almost 10 times more energy for the body to convert excess sugar into fat than it does to just store excess fat: "If you have 100 extra calories in fat floating in your bloodstream, fat cells can store it using only 2.5 calories of energy. On the other hand, if you have 100 extra calories in glucose floating in your bloodstream, it takes 23 calories of energy to convert the glucose into fat" (Freudenrich, 2000, para. 7).

However, fat is not as readily stored without insulin, so be warned: eating the two together (carbs and fat) seems to be a recipe for accelerated fat storage, and your body's instincts know this. This is why cakes, biscuits and chocolate taste so nice to us. Your instincts understand that this combination of macronutrients will facilitate fat storage as quickly as possible, thus increasing your chances of surviving the next imminent food shortage – ie the winter it believes is coming, based on the naturally-occurring autumnal formula that just passed your lips.

Key Point: insulin is the trigger that tells the body's cells to deal with the sugar currently circulating in your blood stream. All your body cares about is having enough energy available for the now, and, if it has, it will store as much of the excess it can for use later on. At the end of the day, we are a type of machine, a biological, self-healing, self-assembling machine that uses the energy available to it, supplied by nature. If you eat carbs, your body will yell "Yippee!!!" and thrive on the sugary energy available (think of kids going wild at a party). It will utilise and store as much of this short-term energy immediately, in the form of glycogen in your liver and muscles, and it will convert the excess to fat. To make matters worse, if you eat fat at the same time as this sugar excess, it will store the fat in your cells more readily, because the insulin response is signalling your cells to store fat. All of this combined with your natural instincts to gorge further means you don't stand a chance if you are prone to putting on weight quickly.

On the other hand, if you had eaten just fat and protein together, with fewer carbs, your body will not have as much sugar energy available and will not produce such a pronounced insulin response. Thus, the body is more likely to utilise the fat in the blood stream as a source of energy and for body function, rather than storing it for future use. There will be a mild insulin response, which will allow the body to store some of the nutrients, in particular the protein itself. Also, the natural instincts to gorge will not be triggered, and you will be more satiated by the food you've just eaten.

Some nutritionists and dieticians argue that it doesn't matter what you eat if you want to lose weight, once you create a calorie deficit. It is true that if you expend more calories than you consume you will lose weight. However, creating a calorie deficit can be misery. There seems to be an easier way.

As discussed, there is research showing that lower-carb diets cause increased metabolism (Ebbeling et al., 2012, p. 2627) – perhaps the furnace may simply burn hotter as a whole, when burning fat. Also, there is much research showing that lower-carb diets result in greater weight loss and yield significant health benefits too (Gunnars, 2013).

Body Types

There are various body types, some of which seem to handle carbs in an incredible way. Some people can seemingly eat anything and not put on any weight, but often struggle to put on muscle, too. So, what is different about people who can put up weight? Genetics? Perhaps their ancestral heritage, and what foods were available to their branch of the human story.

Very little theoretical research has been done in this subject. However, the people with the greatest practical experience in this area are bodybuilders, who have, through years of experimentation, figured out the foods that best suit different body types. There are three main body types: ectomorph, mesomorph and endomorph.

The ectomorph is of slim build and finds it difficult to put on body fat and muscle, and can eat a high quantity of carbs.

The mesomorph has a stronger build than the ectomorph and finds it easier to put on muscle, but does not pile on body fat easily. They can eat a moderate amount of carbs.

The endomorph has the thickest build and can put on body fat and muscle easily and should limit the carbs they eat.

Some good links on suitable macronutrient ratios for body types can be found at the following URL:

www.donteatforwinter.com/book-links

I have to eat like an endomorph because, from experience I have found that I have only lost weight dramatically on controlled carb diets. Initially, I didn't understand why this was. I tried many calorie-counting diets but always found them difficult and put the weight back on as soon as I stopped, because I wasn't managing the carb aspect of my diet.

Bodybuilders use carb cutting and carb cycling as techniques for losing body fat before a competition, but typically they never cut protein and fat during this critical phase, so as to limit muscle loss (which is somewhat inevitable as part of a serious cut) and to maintain health and energy. This got me asking questions such as: Why are carbs (or lack thereof) the best way for these athletes to get in shape? Is it to do with the insulin response? If so, what is it about insulin response that causes us to retain and store excess fat and sugar? Then I started hypothesising on the fundamental reason and asked myself the question:

Why would nature want us to get fat? It was then that I had the Eureka moment ...

Nature wants us to get fat in autumn to protect us from winter!

As stated earlier, I noticed that nature develops all these sweet and starchy carbs in autumn, in order to fatten us up for the bleak, barren and bitter winter ahead. Bodybuilders discovered this practically, through trial and error, and cut autumnal foods to achieve very low levels of bodyfat, whilst maintaining lean muscle mass.

We Can All Learn from Diabetics

There are two main types of diabetes: type 1 and type 2. Both conditions are rooted in the body's inability to either produce insulin or deal with it correctly. Type 1 is an auto-immune disease where the body's immune system attacks the pancreas, essentially destroying its ability to produce insulin. Type 2 diabetes comes about after the body's cells become overly insulin resistant.

Type 1 diabetics must inject themselves with insulin after every meal, so that their cells can absorb the sugar that is circulating through their blood stream. The amount of insulin required varies from person to person, but it is directly related to the quantity of carbs eaten. Carb counting is the typical method for estimating the insulin dose, but recent research suggests that the Glycemic Load (GL) trumps this as a more accurate way of estimating dosage (Bao et al., 2011, p. 984).

The GL of a carb serving is related to its GI. The GL is calculated by measuring the grams of carb in the serving, and multiplying it by the GI of the food, and then dividing the total by 100. A score of 10 or below has a low GL, 20 or higher is a high GL. For example, a small bottle of a glucose drink might have a GL of 40, whereas an apple has a GL of 5. Some useful links regarding GI and GL can be found here: www.donteatforwinter.com/book-links/

Key Point: low GI labelling can sometimes be a bit of a misnomer as something with practically zero calories, such as an onion has a low GI, but so too can carb loaded fibrous autumnal produce. The GL can be a better indication of how quantities of these foods affect our blood sugar levels and the resulting insulin response.

Type 2 diabetics, on the other hand, find that their cells become insulin-resistant and, as a result, the pancreas starts producing more and more insulin in order to try to force the body's cells to absorb sugar from the bloodstream. At some point, the pancreas may give up and no longer produce enough insulin to control blood sugar levels, and thus treatment becomes necessary. Often weight control and exercise can reverse type 2 diabetes and can also be used as ways to control blood sugars for type 1 diabetics.

There is also gestational diabetes, where a pregnant mother goes through a temporary period where cells become insulin resistant and there can be complications, such as a larger than normal infant. Usually, this type of diabetes reverses after the pregnancy.

Insulin-resistance variability is a built-in function of our cells, especially the body's cells. The brain runs almost exclusively on sugar and so it has a low resistance to insulin at all times. The body's cells can turn up or down their resistance depending on various factors.

People who exercise more tend to have cells that are more sensitive to insulin. This can be considered as a type of fitness, as they are more efficient at absorbing glycogen (the muscles' storage form of glucose/sugar), and need to store it more quickly in order to prime their muscles for the next action. People carrying subcutaneous body fat (fat under the skin) tend to have cells that are more insulin resistant. Our bodies traditionally didn't have to deal with the amount of sugar we eat today, at least not all year long. However, we tend to overload that system until it malfunctions and then related health issues ensue. It is truly amazing the punishment our bodies can take before they give up the ghost.

Diabetics must be incredibly careful not to become hyperglycaemic or hypoglycaemic – hyper meaning too much sugar and hypo meaning too little. The brain is the organ most immediately affected by these conditions as it relies on sugar as its main source of energy. Both hypo and hyper are extremely dangerous and can result in drunken-like behaviour, loss of consciousness, weakness, or even coma. There are a multitude of other health issues associated with diabetes, and micromanagement of the condition is required on an hourly basis. It is not a pleasant condition and sufferers and their families encounter a lot of daily worry.

Non-diabetics should realise that both conditions are on the rise. Type 2 diabetes is related to obesity and the over consumption of carbs, in particular refined sugars in modern diets such as sugary fizzy drinks. This all points to the fact that our bodies are not designed to cope with a perpetual bombardment of sugars, which, as discussed, simply isn't natural. During our history, we evolved to cope with the seasons and their produce, and so carbs were not available for most months of the year, giving our pancreas a break. It's no coincidence, therefore, that type 2 diabetes can be managed and even reversed, in many cases, through diet and exercise mimicking how our ancestors would have lived in their natural environment. Our cells seem to become insulin resistant as a natural response to constant bombardment. They can then reset and become sensitive again, when the diet is altered and exercise is introduced.

Type 1 is also on the increase, and scientists think the factors involved in this are environmental, though they are not entirely sure why. They suspect things like lack of vitamins such as D3, amongst other things maybe at the root of it. It might be controversial to suggest, but perhaps one of these factors is the modern diet. At no time in history has there been so much refined, carb-based food available all year around. What if the body's immune system retaliates against its own pancreas because it sees a perpetual bombardment of insulin as an attack? Obviously, type I sufferers have the predisposition towards the condition for some genetic reason, but the trigger is being pulled more often on it. In the same way that other diseases to which a person is predisposed as a result of smoking, drinking alcohol etc, sugar could be a factor here. At the moment, nobody has the full answer.

All Calories are Equal, but Some Calories Are More Equal than Others

A paper entitled "Effects of Dietary Composition on Energy Expenditure During Weight-Loss Maintenance" states: "The results of our study challenge the notion that a calorie is a calorie from a metabolic perspective." The results showed that after weight loss, participants on a very low-carb diet compared with a low-fat diet burned almost 300 calories a day more, "corresponding with the amount of energy typically expended in 1 hour of moderate-intensity physical activity" (Ebbeling et al., 2012, p. 2627).

Aside: personally, I am not a fan of *all out* ketogenic, high fat diets with a very low amount of carb and protein, especially over the long term, however they are very effective for losing weight and seem most effective for increasing metabolism. They can also be used as a treatment for certain medical conditions. I am more in favour of a controlled carb diet, utilising them as a tool to feed the body and mind when needed, and in particular when very active.

If you think about it, our bodies ingest food for three major reasons:

1. Energy (anaerobic, aerobic, brain, etc)
2. Construction and repair (bones, muscle, etc)

3. Function (hormones, immune system, etc)

For energy, we use carbs and fats predominantly, and for construction, repair and function we use fats, proteins, fibre, vitamins and minerals to keep our bodies in tip-top working condition. Obviously, we require water, air and sunlight, too.

From this point of view, all calories are certainly not equal, ie proteins, fats and fibrous foods are far more beneficial to our body health than more starchy and sugary high GI foods, which are, in general, primarily utilised for energy. The former are far more than just energy calories: they contain the building blocks of what we are. Of course, high fibre carbs are important for several reasons too.

Macronutrients and Micronutrients
As stated earlier, there are three types of nutrients the body requires in large quantities, known as macronutrients, ie fat, protein and carbs. These are broken down into fatty acids, amino acids and glucose, respectively, through digestion and used by the body for body repair and functions such as hormone production, constructing bone and muscle and producing energy. Some of the broken-down components are considered essential nutrients, such as the nine essential amino acids in protein (phenylalanine, valine, threonine, tryptophan,

methionine, leucine, isoleucine, lysine, and histidine), and the two essential fatty acids (alpha-linolenic acid, known as ALA, an omega-3, and linoleic acid, an omega-6).

They are called essential nutrients because the body cannot produce them itself, but has to get them from food. Other essential nutrients that the body needs are known as micronutrients, an array of vitamins and minerals required in smaller quantities for cell construction and optimal health.

The word *mineral* can be confusing. It doesn't mean compound minerals, such as crystals, which exist in their thousands of species; it actually means the chemical elements found in the periodic table (atoms) that are required by the human body, except for four of the elements: carbon, hydrogen, oxygen, and nitrogen, which are called non-mineral elements (as they form parts of other compounds such as water). The four non-mineral elements, along with calcium and phosphorous, make up about 99% of the mass of the body: potassium, sodium, chlorine and magnesium bring us up to 99.85%, and the rest, called trace elements account for only about 10 grams of body weight. As many as 29 are suggested to be used by mammals.

Vitamins are vital molecules and are also essential nutrients that again cannot be created by the human body, so they need to be ingested through dietary intake. These act as enzymatic cofactors to assist biochemical transformations; metabolic regulators to assist catabolism or anabolism; and antioxidants to prevent damage to cells by mopping up free radicals.

For more information regarding macro and micronutrients, including essential vitamins and minerals, visit the following link, which includes links to recommended daily allowances, vitamins their functions and foods in which they can be found, etc.

www.donteatforwinter.com/book-links

Here is a quick summary table of macro and micro-nutrients, their function and some foods in which they are found.

Table 1 – Macronutrients

Nutrient	Function	Food
Macronutrients (bulk of diet)		
Fat Mono-unsaturated and poly-unsaturated fats are considered good fats and help to keep heart healthy. Obtained from plants and fish	1. Provides immediate aerobic energy when broken down through digestion 2. Excess can be stored easily as backup energy in fat cells (especially when cells are triggered by insulin) 3. Supports cell function	Meat Eggs Fish Poultry Nuts Avocado Seeds Dairy Oils

Saturated fats are solid at room temperature, eg lard, coconut oil, butter Trans/saturated, hydrogenated fats are modified and considered least healthy	4. Subcutaneous (under skin) fat stores can help to keep body insulated 5. Helps absorb micronutrients (vitamins A, D, E and K) 6. Helps produce important hormones 7. Can be used partially by brain and muscles as a substitute for glucose in a fasted state (ketosis)	
Protein Nine essential amino acids must be consumed (body cannot produce) Non-essential can be created by the body Conditional: needed during times of illness	1. Broken down into amino acids through digestion 2. Essential for building and maintaining muscle mass 3. Repairs cells 4. Helps make new cells 5. Critical for growth 6. Can be used to convert to fuel for brain, along with fat during fasted state	Eggs Meat Fish Poultry Veg Nuts Seeds Soya Milk (whey)
Carbs Foods and drinks containing starch or various forms of sugar. All are converted to glucose to circulate through bloodstream Fibrous carbs are considered better, as they provide a much slower release of sugar and contain other nutrients and fibre	1. Primarily provides energy for brain and muscles, after being converted to glucose through digestion 2. Stored in muscles and liver as glycogen for brain and muscle energy (anaerobic) 3. Sugar in blood can be used in conjunction with oxygen for aerobic energy 4. Excess can be converted to fat for storage in fat cells 5. Fibrous carbs help with slowing digestion (lower GI). Also, help to pass waste and can lower cholesterol	Grain Beets Potato Veg Fruit Honey Syrups Pasta Pastry Bread Sugars

Table 2 – Essential Micronutrients - Vitamins

Essential Micronutrients – Vitamins

Vitamin A (Retinol, retinal, retinoic acid, beta-carotine)	Important for eye health, growth and immune system	Carrots Squashes Fish Liver
Vitamin B1 (Thiamin)	Important for entire body, nervous system circulation etc. A critical vitamin	Pork Fish Seeds Cereals Nuts Legumes
Vitamin B2 (Riboflavin)	The vitamin that makes urine bright yellow. Activates other vitamins. Important for eye health, energy production, migraine prevention. Deficiency can cause swollen lips, scaly rash on mouth, nose, and genitals, and a form of anaemia. Deficiency during pregnancy can cause heart defects in foetus.	Dairy Eggs Leafy veg Kidneys Legumes Mushrooms Almonds
Vitamin B3 (Niacin)	Used in fat catabolism. Treats high cholesterol. Deficiency can cause nausea, skin and mouth lesions, anaemia, headaches, and tiredness. Can treat heart disease for those not on statins	Chicken Beef Venison Tuna Salmon Avocado Broccoli Nuts Legumes Beer ☺
Vitamin B5 (Pantothenic acid)	Energy production. Deficiency can cause numbness, cramps, irritability, hypoglycaemia. It is rare to be deficient in this vitamin	Mushroom Liver Egg yolks Sunflower Wholegrain
Vitamin B6 (Pyridoxal,	Energy production. Deficiency can cause dermatitis-like eruption, ulceration, sores on side of mouth,	Pork Turkey Beef

pyridoxine, pyridoxamine)	conjunctivitis, impaired glucose tolerance	Bananas Chickpeas Potatoes Pistachios
Vitamin B7 (Biotin, formerly vitamin H)	Metabolism of fats and protein. Deficiency can cause hair thinning, brittle nails, rash on face, depression, tingling of hands and feet	Peanuts Leafy veg Egg yoke Liver
Vitamin B9 (Folic acid, folate, folacin)	Important during pregnancy to prevent birth defects. Important for male and fertility. Works with iron and B12. Reduces rates of stroke and heart disease. Deficiency can cause depression, grey hair, mouth sores	Avocado Beetroot Spinach Liver Yeast Asparagus Sprouts
Vitamin B12 (Cobalamin)	Important for brain and nervous system function, red blood cell production. Deficiency can cause depression, fatigue, poor memory, mania and psychosis. Rare in plant sources. Can manifest as anaemia (low red blood cell count)	Meat Fish Dairy
Choline	Reduces the risk of neural tube defects (eg spina bifida), fatty liver disease (alcohol related, obesity related), and other pathologies	Cauliflower Broccoli Cod Soya beans Brown rice Eggs Beef Liver Tofu
Vitamin C (Ascorbic acid)	Utilised by immune system, powerful anti-oxidant. Deficiency leads to scurvy (spongey gums and mouth sores), which is extremely rare today	Blackcurrant Kiwi fruit Broccoli Strawberry Oranges
Vitamin D3 (Cholecalciferol)	Helps with absorption of calcium and aids immune system. Deficiency impairs bone mineralization, which leads to bone-softening diseases. Very	Salmon Mackerel Cod Lichen

	important for children and elderly people. Direct sunlight converts cholesterol to vitamin D	Alfalfa Mushrooms Sunlight
Vitamin E (Alpha-tocopherol)	Powerful anti-oxidant, used in smooth muscle growth. Has a role in eye and neurological functions. Not beneficial to supplement with if healthy	Oils Sunflower Almond Olive Peanut
Vitamin K (phylloquinone, menadione)	Used in synthesis of proteins and absorption of calcium. Found in base form (K1) in green leafy plants due to photosynthesis. Low levels of vitamin K impairs blood coagulation, causing bleeds such as nose bleeds and heavy menstrual bleeding. Deficiency also may lead to weakened bones (osteoporosis) and calcification of arteries, leading to coronary heart disease	Kale Spinach Broccoli Sprouts
Note: Vitamins A, D, E and K are fat soluble. All others are water soluble		

Table 3 – Essential Micronutrients - Minerals

Essential Micronutrients – Minerals		
Calcium	Needed for muscle, heart and digestive system, bones, teeth, blood. Vitamin D is needed to absorb calcium	Dairy Nuts Seeds Quinoa
Chlorine/Chloride	Needed for stomach acid, cell function, combined with sodium and potassium	Salts
Chromium	Blood sugar control. Helps transport glucose into cells	Bran Wholegrain Broccoli
Cobalt	Works with vitamin B12. Important for healthy red blood cells	Same as B12
Copper	Iron metabolism, creation of red blood cells	Liver Shellfish Nuts

		Seeds
		Wholegrain
		Beans
Iodine	Required for thyroid function. Regulates body temperature and assists muscle function. Important for reproduction, and growth	Seaweed Iodized salt Supplement
Iron	Helps transport oxygen throughout body via red blood cells and muscle cells. Supports biochemical reactions for making amino acids, collagen hormones, etc	Meat Eggs Berries Veg
Magnesium	Required for muscle contraction (with calcium) and helps build bones and teeth	Spinach Broccoli Seeds Milk
Manganese	Helps to build bones and metabolise amino acids and carbs	Nuts, Legumes Wholegrain
Molybdenum	Part of many enzymes. Important for prevention of neurological damage in infants	Legumes Nuts Wholegrain Milk
Phosphorus	Helps to build bones and teeth, and assists in the transport of nutrients in and out of cells	Dairy Meat Fish Eggs Peas Broccoli Almonds
Potassium	Electrolyte, fluid balance. Works with sodium in muscle contraction, regulates heart, lowers blood pressure	Avocado Spinach Coconut-Water Meat Banana
Selenium	Antioxidant. Assists thyroid function	Brazil nuts Beef Turkey Sardines

Sodium	Electrolyte, fluid balance, works with potassium in muscle contraction, regulates heart, can raise blood pressure	Salt (use natural salts)
Sulphur	For healthy hair, skin and nails	Meat Fish Nuts Legumes
Zinc	Immune system support, taste, smell, and healing	Oysters Nuts Seeds Cocao

Key Take Home Point: you don't need to remember all of the above. Try to eat a balanced diet containing lots of colour, including veg, fruits and berries; good sources of protein and fat such as meat, poultry fish, eggs, nuts, seeds, avocados and olive oil; and fibre-rich carbs such as wholegrains, and you will cover most bases. It's always an idea to have a good multi-vitamin and mineral supplement to make sure you have the recommended daily amounts of everything you require to stay healthy. Natural salts, such as sea and rock salt, may also be better than common table salt, as they contain trace minerals too. Remember, if supplementing, to take vitamins A, D, E and K with meals containing fat, as they are fat soluble.

Macronutrient Breakdown (Literally!)

Let's break the macronutrients down in more detail (just as your body does):

Fat Facts

According to the American Heart Association: "Dietary fats are essential to *give your body energy* and to *support cell growth*. They also help to protect your organs and *help keep your body warm*. Fats help your body *absorb some nutrients* and *produce important hormones*, too" (American Heart Organisation, 2017, p. 101, my emphasis).

There are four main types of fat:

1. **Trans fat:** hydrogenated fat to facilitate cooking and preserving (found in fast food, biscuits, artificial spreads)
2. **Saturated fat:** solid fats like butter, coconut oil and lard from farmed animals
3. **Monounsaturated fats (MUFAs):** fat in plants, seeds, nuts and wild game
4. **Polyunsaturated fats (PUFAs):** found in fish, plants, seeds and nuts and wild game. Includes important Omega-3s, such as the essential fatty acid ALA

Two of these fats are *traditionally* considered harmful, ie saturated fat and trans fat. Saturated fat comes from meat, dairy and some plants and is generally solid at room temperature (for example lard, butter, coconut oil). Trans fats, otherwise known as partially hydrogenated fats, are oils that are artificially modified to keep them from spoiling. This often makes them more suitable for cheaper, processed foods and fast foods. Both are traditionally said to cause high cholesterol, which may lead to cardiovascular disease. There is new evidence, however, suggesting that saturated fat is not as dangerous as once suggested, especially if consumed in moderation. Trans fats are still considered the least healthy type of fat.

The other two types of fat are considered healthy fats, ie monounsaturated fats (MUFAs) and polyunsaturated fats (PUFAs), of which Omega-3s are particularly important for heart health, as they actively lower *bad* cholesterol. MUFAs are found in a variety of plant-based foods such as avocados, olives, olive oil, rapeseed oil, almonds, cashews, hazelnuts, peanuts, pistachios and spreads made from these nuts. PUFAs are a type of fat found in oily fish such as salmon, tuna, trout, mackerel, sardines and herring, and plants such as sesame, soya, flaxseed, chia seeds, pine nuts, sesame seeds, sunflower seeds, and walnuts. Wild game can also be a better source of fat from meat as it often contains a higher ratio of healthy fats.

There is more to fat, however, as it is also very important for your production of hormones (endocrine system) and so eating adequate amounts of fat in your diet is crucial to regulating metabolism, sexual function, sleep and mood, among other things. Fats help to carry some vitamins (ADEK) into the body too, so it is a good idea, if you are supplementing with fat soluble vitamins, to take them with a meal containing fat.

According to the US National Library of Medicine:

"You also need fat to keep your skin and hair healthy. Fat also helps you absorb vitamins A, D, E, and K, the so-called fat-soluble vitamins. Fat also fills your fat cells and *insulates your body to help keep you warm*" (Martin et al., 2016, para. 4, my emphasis)

According to the Institute of Medicine (US), the acceptable amount of fat consumed per day depends on age and gender. However, somewhere between 20% to 35% is acceptable for most adults. In the proverbial 2,000 calorie diet, this equates to about 400–700 calories or 44–77 grams as one gram of fat is equal to about nine calories. Links to this data can be found at the following URL:

www.donteatforwinter.com/book-links

Key Point: so many people opt for low-fat foods now, which are generally high in sugar and heavily processed, because of the fear factor about heart disease (which is now under question). Fat is totally essential for a healthy body, though, it is advisable to *avoid trans fats*. Natural, saturated fats should be consumed in moderation, and the focus should be on consuming most fats in the form of mono- and polyunsaturated fats because of their positive effects on health and their role in supporting other bodily functions. Eating these types of fats can help to prevent heart disease and can lower cholesterol.

The Pros of Protein

According to the US National Library of Medicine: "you need protein in your diet to *help your body repair cells* and *make new ones*. Protein is also important for *growth and development* in children, teens, and pregnant women" (Wax et al., 2017, para. 2, my emphasis)

Protein is broken down during digestion into amino acids. Amino acids are found in staples such as meats, fish, and eggs and in plants such as nuts, legumes, and some grains.

There are three main types of amino acid:

1. Essential: these are not produced by the body and must be acquired from external sources
2. Non-essential: made by the body from essential amino acids and so are not necessary to consume directly
3. Conditional: required during times of illness

Some healthy sources of protein from staples include: chicken, turkey, beef, pork, salmon, cod, eggs. Other good sources of protein from plants include: legumes such as beans, peas and, nuts such as peanuts, walnuts, almonds, brazils, seeds and soy.

Tip for Vegans and Vegetarians: it's worth noting that if you eat a diet of plant produce, you cannot get all essential amino acids from just one source, and so you must eat a combination of foods to get the full spectrum. Traditionally it was suggested that these were required during one sitting, but now it is thought that it is good enough to ingest the spectrum throughout the course of the day. However, it's no harm to try to get them all as close together as possible.

Meat, fish and eggs, however, do contain the full spectrum of amino acids. Another source of protein of course is dairy. However, many people are lactose intolerant and dairy can sometimes be over-processed, so watch the ingredients.

Protein is particularly important, if you are active, for the repair, maintenance and growth of muscle tissues, which is why athletes sometimes supplement their diet with protein shakes. This supplementation is often used for economic reasons, as eating a lot of meat, fish and eggs can be much more expensive than a scoop of protein powder in a shake.

Supplementation should not result in the replacement of natural foods, but may be used in conjunction with them, when necessary. If you do supplement with protein, try to use one with few added sugars and ingredients. You could consider using berries, fruit, veg, nuts, seeds, wholegrains and other ingredients to add natural carbs, fats, flavour, fibre, vitamins and minerals to your smoothies, depending on your requirements.

The acceptable amount of protein per day (according to the Institute of Medicine) depends on your level of activity, but somewhere between 10% and 35% of an adult diet is recommended. This equates to around 200–700 calories of a 2,000-calorie diet, or 50–175 grams per day (one gram of protein is equal to about four calories). A measure of 175 grams is a large amount and would be more suitable for a hard-working athlete, for example. However, even a sedentary person should ensure adequate protein is taken to help to maintain muscle mass. The downside of protein is that it can be tough for your kidneys to process, especially if you don't need it for repairing torn muscle fibres. Links to this data can be found at the following URL: www.donteatforwinter.com/book-links

Carbohydrates

Carbs are basically various forms of sugar. There are saccharides (simple sugars), disaccharides (naturally occurring sugars) and polysaccharides (starches). Technically, fibre can be counted as a carb, and is typically found in the flesh and skin of carb sources. However, we deal with it separately, as fibre is not converted to sugar by the body.

Most people do not understand how many foods are essentially sugars, even if they don't taste particularly sweet. For example, potatoes, rice, pasta, bread, root veg like turnips, and milk contain comparatively high amounts of sugar.

Our bodies' immediate energy source is sugar, so we need it to be available to our brain and body. According to Berg et al.:

"The brain lacks fuel stores and hence requires a continuous supply of glucose. It consumes about 120 g daily, which corresponds to an energy input of about 420 kcal (1760 kJ), accounting for some 60% of the utilization of glucose by the whole body in the resting state" (2002, p. 30.2).

The Institute of Medicine suggest approximately 130 grams at a minimum, which equates to about 520 calories from carbs at a minimum, per day. The Acceptable Macronutrient Distribution Range (AMDR) for carb is 45 to 65% of total calories. At 45%, this means that our body's basic allowance for carbs, in the standard 2,000-calory reference diet, is approximately 900 calories or 360 grams. This is a surplus of 480 calories over brain requirement for your body's muscles to use for energy purposes.

When inactive, our bodies can use fatty acids as a major fuel source: "In resting muscle, fatty acids are the major fuel, meeting 85% of the energy needs." (Berg et al., 2002, p. 30.2).

Therefore, I would suggest that 45% of a 2,000-calorie diet is more than ample for energy needs in this case, especially if you are sedentary. However, if you *are* active, your body may require more sugar energy, both anaerobically and aerobically (explained later), and you will definitely require more carbs than if you were sedentary all day. In the case of physical labourers or athletes, you could approach, or even potentially exceed, the upper limit of 65%, depending on the type, duration and intensity of the activity being supported.

The main problem today, however, is that we eat far too many carbs for our daily sugar-based energy requirements. Fat and protein are generally used by your body to maintain it, repairing muscles, skin, hair, producing hormones and so on. Carbs, on the other hand, are consumed mainly for a sole purpose: energy.

Of course, some carbs sources are loaded with vitamins, minerals and fibre, and all of this is fantastic, but the message of The DEFoW Diet is simple:

Eat sugary and starchy carbs, ie autumnal foods, in moderation and based on your daily energy requirements, because any excess of this macronutrient, in particular, results in an energy surplus, and thus triggers fat storage.

Key Point: when the body receives carbs, it releases sugar into the blood stream as glucose. Some of this sugar is used for immediate energy purposes (like using a phone when it is plugged in). The body will convert glucose to glycogen and will store as much as possible in muscles (for anaerobic energy) and liver (for backup supply to maintain blood sugar levels), like a short-term backup battery for demanding near-future energy needs. Any excess after this will be converted to fat and stored in fat cells as a backup battery for longer-term respiratory energy needs.

So, if your job includes strenuous manual labour, or you work out intensively in the gym or with your sport, you will need more than the minimum supply of carbs. If you sit in an office at a computer all day, and do nothing but sit on the couch when you get home, then you just need the minimum required by your brain and body.

Whether you are sedentary or active, if you have an excess intake of carbs you will encourage fat storage. Therefore, in so far as is possible, you should only consume the exact amount of carbs required by your body and brain. The rest of your calories should come from proteins, fats and fibrous low GI spring and summer foods, in order to generate the best version of you, as you produce new cells.

Fibre

It is important to understand the role of fibre in your diet, and where to get it. In the past, people ate a wide variety of wild foods that were rich in fibre, but these days, over-processing has taken a lot of good out of the foods. Fibre is available through plant produce: generally it is found in the skin and flesh of fruits, veg, nuts and seeds and the bran of grains, etc. There are two types of fibre: soluble and non-soluble.

Non-soluble fibre can assist with increasing the volume and speedy passing of waste from your body, and is typically found in the bran of grains. Soluble fibre, on the other hand, is found in the flesh of fruit and vegetables, and helps to lower cholesterol.

Fibrous foods are more filling and the non-soluble and thus non-digestible kind passes all the way through your body, carrying other toxins with them. So, when you eat them you are not getting any calories from them, but you are filling your stomach and helping your body to detoxify.

Fibre can also slow the digestion of carbs, lowering the GI of the food. Typically, fibrous carbs are known as "good carbs" as they are typically full of nutrients and are digested at a natural pace.

Water and Electrolytes

It is important that we don't forget the most important essential nutrient, which is of course water. You must drink ample amounts of water each day for optimal health, to flush out toxins, and to keep yourself hydrated, so that your body and brain work well. Get a good quality water supply. There is a debate about chemicals in tap water: some are necessary to kill bacteria in the supply; others are there in some jurisdictions for medication purposes, for example fluoride, which is present to prevent dental caries/cavities.

This book is not about fearmongering, so if you're worried about chemicals in your supply (you'll know if it tastes bad or a dog won't drink it) the solution is a good home filtration system, which is relatively inexpensive these days. This can remove most chemicals, including fluoride (for example reverse osmosis) if you are worried about them. Alternatively, you could choose to drink bottled water, but be careful of the type of plastic it's stored in. Glass is always better.

If you sweat a lot because of training, or get a bout of diarrhoea, you will lose a lot of salts and minerals known as electrolytes, including: sodium, chloride, potassium, magnesium, calcium, bicarbonate and phosphate. Under these circumstances, it is important to replenish these, in the right balance, through supplementation (for example electrolyte drinks or rehydration sachets), as they are critical for many functions within the body, including muscle contraction (preventing cramp), maintaining blood pressure, nervous system, and cell function. Without these, you will be very weak. All athletes should make sure they are well hydrated with electrolytes before, during and when recovering from exercise.

Sunlight

Sunlight is not technically an essential nutrient, but it does have an effect on our bodies. UV light interacts with the cholesterol that exists just under our skin, in order to synthesize vitamin D3. Vitamin D is critical for healthy bones and plays other important roles in our bodies. So, try to and spend some time every day with sunlight shining on your skin, but being mindful of avoiding sunburn (don't stay exposed too long). If you cannot get adequate sunlight, consider supplementing during the darkest months of winter with a vitamin D3 supplement. Read the label carefully and do not overdose on D3, as it can cause a build-up of calcium in your body. Sunlight is good for wellbeing in general, so enjoy it when it's available.

Air

Good air is also very important to us, and modern studies show that polluted air is almost as bad for us as smoking. In your home, ensure there is no carbon monoxide or radon gas, and that ventilation is good; and if city air quality is particularly bad in your area, consider an air purification system.

When you can, try to get out of the city to areas to where the air is good – the coast, the mountains, forests, etc. Go out into to nature and enjoy the air and sunlight, and why not ground your feet in the dirt and splash in the water to experience life the way we are meant to!

If you smoke, try to quit, and if you cannot quit, consider some alternative means of supplying nicotine that doesn't put as many harmful chemicals, like tar, into your lungs. Vaping seems to be a safer alternative to smoking, though more research needs to be done to confirm this. Public Health England published a report in 2015 suggesting that e-cigarettes are 95% safer than cigarette smoking (para. 1).

Earth, Water, Wind, Fire

A good way to remember the importance of these nutrients is the classical elements, earth wind, water, and fire.

- Fire is the sun – without heat we die instantly.
- Wind is air – without air we die in seconds.
- Water is hydration – without it we die in days.
- Earth is the essential nutrients – without these we die in weeks, but without any we would never have existed in the first place.

Why you <u>Shouldn't</u> Eat for Winter

Here are some traditional reasons why autumnal foods make you gain weight:

1. Autumnal foods are plentiful in supply and require less work to gather. If you have a more sedentary lifestyle, you'll find that these extra calories create a large energy surplus where the excess is converted to fat.

2. According to the National Sleep Foundation, carb-rich meals make tryptophan more available to the brain (if eaten with protein in particular), making you feel drowsy (Davilla, para. 2). Drowsy means more rest, which means less calories burnt off and more fat will be stored.

3. According to the same article large meals, especially carb meals can also accentuate the post lunch dip (Davilla, 2017, para. 4). Autumnal foods make you lethargic, making you less likely to want to do work and therefore burn as many calories resulting in more fat being stored.

4. High GI foods mean more sugar highs and lows. The lows also make you feel tired and less likely to want to do anything (except eat more to compensate), and so more calories are eaten, fewer calories are burnt and more fat is stored as a result.

5. According to a study (Lennerz et al., 2013, p. 1), sugar is addictive, making us want to eat more than we normally would, encouraging excess energy supply and thus more fat storage. These sorts of instincts are present in squirrels and hibernating animals, which we share the planet with. Nature has given us similar primal urges to facilitate our survival. When triggered, we are overcome with an overwhelming urge to gorge, causing a large surplus of energy which encourages fat storage.

6. The conversion of carbs or protein into fat is 10 times less efficient than simply storing fat in a fat cell. This is particularly the case if an insulin response has been triggered through the consumption of large quantities of high GI

foods. If there is no insulin response, the body will utilise the fat eaten for its immediate functional and energy needs. Eating carbs and fat together cause a large energy surplus, along with an insulin response, and the body has no choice to but store that excess energy for future use in the form of fat.

7. Research has shown that people who eat low-fat diets tend to lose less weight than people on low-carb diets. People on low-carb, high-fat diets also see an increase in metabolism and may burn up to 300 more calories per day.

There is an argument as to whether the insulin response has anything to do with weight gain/loss, and many suggest it is simply calorie surplus/deficit that causes weight gain/loss. Even if this is the case, the first five points above still apply, and therefore the logic of not eating for winter is still valid. By not eating for winter, you will feel more energetic and feel more satiated by your food, meaning you will use more calories and, potentially, eat less, causing a daily calorie deficit.

If the sixth and seventh points regarding insulin and metabolism are also true, life may be made a lot easier for anyone prone to storing fat. Eating foods at certain times, and in particular, in certain combinations, may reduce the need for torturous calorie-restricting diets.

I believe this is the case and I am a walking example that it works. I was prone to putting on weight before eating this way, but even loosely sticking to the diet has me at, or close to, my ideal weight without trying too much.

Human Energy Systems

In order to understand how your body burns fat, you must first understand the basics of the human energy systems. Essentially there are two main energy systems: anaerobic and aerobic. The anaerobic system does not require oxygen to operate, whereas the aerobic system does. You know you are working aerobically if you are breathing hard and your heart is pumping faster than normal (of course you are always working somewhat aerobically, even at rest).

The anaerobic system runs off two forms of instant energy that do not require oxygen to work. Our muscles use a molecule called ATP (Adenosine Tri-Phosphate) to contract and move. We store a very small amount of ATP for instant actions like jumping out of the way of danger. This store is refilled once used by the next system, the glycolytic system. This system uses the glycogen (sugar) stored in muscles to produce more ATP. Both of these systems are non-oxidative, ie they don't require oxygen pumped from heart and lungs to operate. The drawback of these two systems is that they deplete quickly and need to be restored. A 100-meter sprint would draw hugely from the ATP and glycogen stores of an athlete and they would start relying on the oxidative or aerobic system if they were to continue running.

The oxidative system or aerobic system uses oxygen combined with either sugar (glycogen) or fat (glycerol and fatty acids) to produce ATP. It takes longer to create ATP from fatty acids so, typically, higher-intensity aerobic activities require more glucose to be available in the bloodstream, which is supplied through your stomach. If you run out of glucose you won't last long performing strenuous work, though long-distance endurance athletes can utilise fat as source of energy. Your body is extremely efficient at providing muscles with energy from fat when at rest or working at a modest pace. In fact, 85% of their energy comes from fat during rest (Berg et al., 2002, p. 30.2). In contrast, when working really hard, most of their energy comes from sugar.

It is only important to have a high-level understanding of this to know that under normal circumstances, *the only system that burns fat is your oxidative/aerobic system*, and it is at its *most efficient while you rest* and when your blood sugars are normal.

The single best way to burn fat is by resting in a somewhat fasted state. You can super charge your fat-burning rate while resting through exercise. If, for example, you do a weights session in the gym, you will burn more fat while you rest than you otherwise would have. This is because of the adaption, recovery and repair work your body needs to do after the exercise session raises your metabolism and you will burn more calories at rest. For this reason, if your goal is to lose body fat, you should always include an exercise regime (you should anyway for general fitness and health to improve your quality of life) as part of a weight loss programme.

It's worth noting that a really tough aerobic session that gets your heart close to its maximum *will not burn significant fat* while you are in the gym. It will also make you feel really bad if you haven't loaded up on enough carbs before it. You must give your body an ample amount of carbs pre-workout in order to have the energy it needs available during a tough session. If you measure this carefully and don't overdo it, when sugar levels quickly revert back to normal after exercise, you will begin burning fat at an accelerated rate while you rest.

There is one more energy draw in the human body, and that is the human brain. The brain requires roughly 420 calories of sugar energy a day, which is actually 60% of the body's total glucose requirement at rest (Berg et al., 2002. p. 230.2).

Aside: people on very low-carb diets do switch to burning fat almost exclusively after some time, as the fat takes on the behaviour of glucose. These diets are known as ketogenic diets, and are not suitable for most ordinary people seeking to lose weight. They can be very effective in treating people with certain medical conditions such as epilepsy and diabetes. However, under a state of ketosis, your body may start breaking down your muscle tissue to create supplementary glucose, primarily for your brain (you couldn't do much without this vital organ). In essence, your body thinks you are starving and it does what it does best, survive!

In simple terms, I think of my body as a vehicle, made of flesh and bones instead of metal and rubber. All vehicles require fuel. When I think of food, I see carbs and fats as fuels for my engine (movement), and fibres, fats and proteins as tools and materials for the mechanics (our cells) to use to keep the machine in tip-top condition. Carbs are like rocket fuel, when used anaerobically, and like high-octane petrol when used aerobically. Fats, on the other hand, are more like a highly efficient, slow burning, reliable diesel fuel for our aerobic system. When lots of excess fuel is supplied to the mechanics, they will store the extra fuel in the boot and back seats (in our fat cells), which weigh down the vehicle, so it's important, for efficiency, to just have enough fuel in the tank for the journey at hand.

Carb for Life

It is crucial to fuel your body correctly for your lifestyle. If you are a physical labourer, you may require a lot more carbs than someone who works at a desk on a computer. If you are inactive, you will still need some carbs for your brain to function well, but you will obviously require a lot fewer than someone with a more physical job because your body does not have the same energy requirements. As stated previously, the brain requires around 420 calories from carbs a day and your body requires about the same again (if you are sedentary). If you work in a physical job, your requirement for sugar will be much larger and so you need to get a handle on how many calories you burn per hour and top up your carb intake accordingly.

If you go to the gym after work and, in particular, if it's a very intense session (for example a 45-minute circuit class), you will certainly need supplementary carbs to fuel both your anaerobic and aerobic systems and to keep your glycogen stores topped up and your blood sugars elevated for immediate aerobic use. In this case, you might need a more instant supply of sugar (higher-GI foods). If you do a longer, slow and steady cardio session, controlling heart and breathing, a more slowly digested carb (lower GI with a higher carb content) source may suit better to keep you going for a longer period of time. For a heavy weights session, you will need ample sugar to keep refilling your muscles glycogen stores, so again carbs are required for this. Therefore, you must tailor your diet based on your activity. But remember, the bulk of fat burning mainly happens afterwards, when you rest and are in a fasted state, and the insulin response to the food has faded.

For most people, I would suggest keeping protein, fat and fibre intakes fairly constant daily, in order to rebuild your body and keep it healthy. The only major variable is carbs, and so you should adjust the amount of these consumed in order to support the physical activities you do. If you do a lot of intense exercise, supplementing protein, vitamins and minerals should also be considered that your body can repair and adapt to the work.

To go back to the analogy of the car, keep the oil (fat and protein) topped up to keep the engine running smoothly, and put enough fuel (carbs) in the tank for the immediate journey ahead. In the case of a very long exercise session, such as a very long walk or hike, where you are continuously working for hours, fat may be an appropriate source of energy along with slow release carbs, especially if you have a low percentage of body fat and are not trying to lose any more weight.

Chapter 5

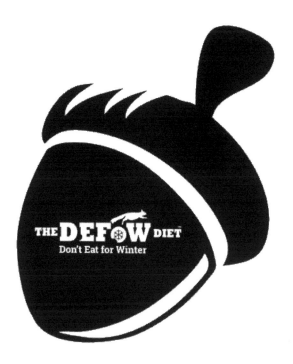

*Unlock Nature's Secret
to Reveal Your True Body*

The DEFoW Diet

After reading all about the macronutrients and their effects on us, and how the energy systems of the body work, we are now finally ready to look at The DEFoW Diet in detail. There are many reasons why this way of eating might be right for you. The term diet has negative connotations, because there have been so many fad diets and so many failed results and rebounds. People tend to bounce back after they reach their goals as the diets were too restrictive or punishing, and their bodies react again through instinct when trigger foods are added back into the diet.

Let's reiterate two key points:

- Foods *harvested in autumn* are designed, by nature, to *facilitate fat storage*, in order to give humans and animals their best chance at *surviving the famine and cold* of winter.
- The fact that *autumnal foods* are so readily available *all year round*, creates a recipe for *perpetual weight gain* in order to prepare us for a *winter that never comes*!

Remember, nature wants to seduce you, through your instincts, into getting fatter in order to protect you and keep you alive. When you eat autumnal foods, these ancient instincts are triggered which encourage fat storage. Your instincts are not aware that the local supermarkets are selling apples and cereals in spring, but if you eat them it will cause the same response in your body that it would have 10,000 years ago, in September. The difference 10,000 years ago was that these foods were only available in autumn, so you didn't have the option to eat them all year around. Nature made the decision for you so you didn't have to. Until now, maybe you weren't aware of this simple fact and why these foods trigger such a response in you. Now that you are aware of this and you know that having these foods available all year around is not natural, it is down to you to apply this knowledge to make the right choices.

The DEFoW Diet simply helps you make the right choices so that you:

- Don't eat foods and combinations that trigger instinctual, addiction like cravings.
- Don't eat food combinations that encourage fat storage.
- Eat a more precise amount of carbs to discourage sugar energy surplus.
- Eat foods that make you feel full so that you don't need to eat as much or as often.
- Feel more energetic and motivated so that you burn more calories every day.

As discussed earlier, if you want to lose weight you should tend towards eating a macro ratio resembling what early humans would have eaten during spring and early summer. If you want to gain weight, then eat a ratio similar to late summer and autumn (the human breast milk macronutrient ratio – remember how fat squirrels got during a mild winter) and if you want to maintain weight, aim for something in between.

The 10 Golden Rules of The DEFoW Diet

Following is a list of 10 guidelines for you to consider. This is The DEFoW Diet version of a Palaeolithic Prescription:

1. Only eat the precise amount of carbs for your body's energy requirements.

2. Avoid eating carbs and fats together to minimise fat deposits and prevent triggering your primal gorge instincts.

3. Eat meals containing fat and protein together, with few to no carbs.

4. When eating meals containing carbs, choose lean protein and avoid fats.

5. Fat is necessary, but eat mainly "good" fats and avoid trans fats.

6. Protein is your muscles' best friend, so eat plenty.

7. Get your fibre, vitamins and minerals from natural sources, where possible, and supplement when necessary.

8. Exercise regularly and support this with diet and rest.

9. Hydrate well.

10. Get out into nature and have fun.

The Golden Rules Explained

1. Only eat the precise amount of carbs for your body's energy requirements (~40% of diet)

Control the amount carbs you eat based on your body's requirements. Remember, the brain requires about 420 calories a day, and at rest your body runs mostly off fat. A good rule of thumb is about 40%, or less, of your calories, especially if you tend to put on weight easily. Control the amount of High GI, starchy and sugary autumnal foods (and avoid processed sugary foods) you eat daily, especially if you are not very active. Eat plenty of low GI, spring/early summer veg to get fibre and vitamins and minerals. Increase the amount of carbs you eat, as necessary, as your fuel source for physical activities such as weight training, high intensity exercise, and tough physical work.

The fewer sugar spikes a day, the more time you will spend burning fat at rest and avoid storing new fat. Your brain and body will utilise the sugar better as your cells become less insulin resistant.

2. Avoid eating carbs and fats together to minimise fat deposits and prevent triggering your primal gorge instincts

When you eat high GI carbs (like refined sugars) your blood sugar levels will rise, which results in a proportional release of insulin. Your body knows that it has ample energy for the now and will switch into storage mode in order to store any excess energy for later. Eating fat, at the same time, compounds the problem as your body will store fat more efficiently at this time. This is the ultimate natural formula for putting on fat (think baby milk). It doesn't mean you should never treat yourself and eat them together, but be aware that this combination is designed by nature to make you gain weight through biochemical processes and will also result in triggering your primal instincts, compounding the problem by encouraging you to gorge. Nature has created you this way to protect you and to prepare you for winter, so don't feel guilty if you succumb to these powerful instincts; but, do understand them and be aware of them. You should also realise that you are being exploited by commercial industries, which have tailored their products to prey on these instincts, and that they rely on your resulting impulse purchases to make profit.

3. Eat meals containing fat and protein together, with few to no carbs

Morning is a good time to eat like this. *This is the spring time of your day*. If your job is at a desk, you will feel full for hours. Avoiding carbs here will prevent an sugar spike and resulting insulin response. As a result your body will be less likely to store fat during this period and continue to burn fat efficiently. Feel free to eat low GI spring/summer produce during this time.

4. When eating meals containing carbs, choose lean protein and avoid fats

During the day, eat lean cuts of meat/fish where possible and get your carbs from plenty of colourful, fibrous, spring/summer veg, leafy greens etc and/or some fruit to give your brain a boost. Avoid large quantities of very starchy carbs in your midday meal, to avoid the mid-afternoon slump. *This is the summer time of your day.* Evening is a great time to eat a slightly larger quantity of some wholegrain, fibrous, starchy carbs, again with leaner cuts of meat and fish – this will help you get a good night sleep. Eat plenty of veg again, such as broccoli, cauliflower etc and avoid high GI foods with this meal, as you want a slow release of sugar into the evening. *This is the autumn time of your day.* If you've exercised in the evening, this will help your body to repair and grow new muscle. By avoiding fat here, you will be less likely to store any excess energy in your fat cells. Remember, it takes a lot more energy for your body to convert carbs into fat than it does to just store fat you've eaten with carbs. If you exercise early in the day, you will want to fuel up with a carb/protein meal with ample time before your session.

5. **Fat is necessary, but eat mainly "good" fats and avoid trans fats (~30-35% of diet)**

Eat poly- and monounsaturated fats mostly from fish, seeds and nuts and avocados, healthy oils, and don't be too concerned about natural saturated fats from meat, eggs, butter and coconut oil. Fats maintain health through supporting your hormones and help to carry vitamins into your body, while polyunsaturated fats (Omega 3 in particular) support heart health and lower cholesterol. *Avoid trans fats, otherwise known as hydrogenated fats, where possible.*

6. **Protein is your muscles' best friend, so eat plenty (~30-35% of daily intake)**

Don't neglect protein if you want to maintain muscle and recover from physical activity. Eat lean protein with carbs to maintain strength. It also tastes good and keeps you satiated. If you are vegan or vegetarian, make sure you eat a variety of foods to get the full spectrum of amino acids. When sick, consider supplementing with L-Glutamine. When training, consider supplementing with protein such as whey, and BCAAs to encourage muscle protein synthesis.

7. **Get your fibre, vitamins and minerals from natural sources, where possible, and supplement when necessary**

Eat pesticide-free fibrous and colourful fruit and veg and plenty of nuts and seeds – the more varied the better. When eating starchy carbs such as grains and rice, and their derived products (breads, pasta etc), eat wholegrain versions, where possible. Eat the skin and flesh of fruit, veg, grain, seeds, etc. Supplement, if you feel you aren't getting the vitamins and minerals you need from your food. A good daily multivitamin tablet is always a good idea, so why not have it with your fat and protein meals, to help to carry the vitamins A, D, E and K into your body?

8. Exercise regularly and support this with diet and rest

When you exercise, you have a larger requirement for carbs and protein. Your body will use sugar for both anaerobic and aerobic energy. By depleting glycogen when you move fast or lift weights, you create a sink for sugar energy and these stores need to be replenished by the sugar supplied to your bloodstream from the food in your stomach. If you do a short, high-intensity workout during the course of an hour-long class in a gym, you will use a lot of sugar too. It is a good idea therefore to fuel up with carbs before training to support you during your training, so that you can give your best, and also afterwards (and potentially during), to restore your muscles glycogen stores so that your body is not stealing the energy required by your brain afterwards. Supporting your training with lean protein (eg egg whites, whey protein etc), before and after, will also help you to build and maintain strong muscles. After training hard, you will burn fat at a faster pace than your otherwise would have while resting. If you are exercising at low intensity over the course of many hours, for example on a long hike or a long-distance run, where your heart rate is moderately higher than normal, you could consider breaking rule 2 by having low GI carbs and fat prior to exercise (for example oats and peanut butter, or brown rice, eggs and oily fish), as your body will utilise both energy systems in this case. Support your recovery with your diet (low GI fibrous carbs, colourful fruit and veg and a good source of protein).

In order to gain from your training, it is also critical that you rest adequately to allow your body to recover. This involves not over-training and getting a decent amount of sleep. By over-training, you will simply undo all your brilliant work.

9. Hydrate well

Make sure your body has enough fluids and electrolytes (salts and minerals) every day. Drink water with every meal, and regularly throughout the day. This is especially important if you sweat a lot because of lifestyle or exercise. Salts help you stay hydrated better and facilitate body functions. Make sure that you get enough potassium from foods, as our diets typically have more than enough sodium-chloride (regular salt) already. If you are adding salt to food, switch to natural salts like sea-salt or rock-salt, as they also contain other useful trace elements. Avoid products containing sodium nitrate and sulphites. If you are exercising, you will find that an electrolyte supplement is a good idea. If exercising very intensely, you will find that the added glucose versions are fine, but if not so intensely, and you've already loaded up on adequate carbs before a session, then low sugar versions are more pragmatic.

10. Get out into nature and have fun

Our bodies need natural sunlight and good air. Our minds and wellbeing are affected positively when we get in touch with nature. Natural sunlight allows our bodies create vitamin D3, which facilitates the absorption of calcium for healthy bones and teeth. If you live in a less sunny country, you must take care to get enough natural light.

Getting away from cities where the air is not polluted is great for you. Feeling the air against your skin and breathing it in deep, while moving about, is energising and will make you feel content.

Nature is fun, great exercise, and where you are meant to be, so get out there and explore it and play with your children, your family and friends. Our world is artificial and the more we get back in touch with our roots, the more likely we are to learn from nature and live by her rules. This is our heritage.

Break the Rules (every now and then)

There is an 11th unwritten rule, and that is to break the rules every now and again. Have a treat, savour the special occasions and let go from time to time. Once it's not too regular, your body will revert to the best version of itself before too long.

What-to-Eat Taxonomy

If you think about the food available in nature, some are constant and others are seasonal. We have staples such as meat, fish, poultry and eggs; then all the seasonal fruit, veg, cereals, tubers, nuts, legumes and seeds; and then semi-natural products such as processed dairy. Of course, then there are highly processed derivatives of these foods designed to taste even more fantastic, so that you keep on buying them through cravings, addiction and impulses.

The Staples: Make Sure You Get Enough of These Daily

Staples are foods that are available all year around. Obviously, fish and seafood varieties are seasonal too, but generally you should eat these every day. Have a portion of each with every main meal:

- Meats
- Fish/seafood
- Poultry
- Eggs

If you're a vegan or vegetarian (an admirable group of people who generally know far more about the benefits of food nutrients than most), try to get essential fats and the full amino acid spectrum from as many natural foods as possible.

Seasonal Carbs: These Should Be Eaten Depending on Your Sugar Energy Requirements

The foods in the table below are your natural seasonal fruit, veg, cereals etc. All of these are healthy and full of natural goodness. You can eat them all: just make sure that you eat the ones in the right-hand column in moderation or, better still, eat them in a meal before/after an activity. Avoid eating them with fats, where possible, but do eat them with lean cuts of meat and fish when eating your carb meal(s). This list is not exhaustive, so if in doubt about a food, you can search for its GI on www.glycemicindex.com

Table 4 – Harvests Spring/Summer vs Autumn/Winter

Spring/Summer Foods (Eat Plenty)	Autumn/Winter Foods (Eat in Moderation)
Veg (practically zero GI)	**Veg**
Cabbage	Marrow
Kale	Pumpkin
Cauliflower	Squashes
Asparagus	Carrots
Brocolli	Parsnips
Leeks	Turnips
Cucumber	Beetroot
Spinach	**Legumes**
Lettuce	Peas, beans and peanuts
Courgettes	**Cereals**
Tomatoes	Corn
Onions	Wheat
Scallions	Oats
	Rice
Berries/fruit (these have some sugars)	**Tubers**
Strawberries	Potatoes
Cherries	Sweet Potatoes
Raspberries	**Sweet Fruits**
Blackcurrants	Apples
Blueberries	Peaches, nectarines and apricots
Rhubarb	Pears
	Plums
	Grapes

Note: You could consider putting on a little weight in winter and eating more of the autumnal foods when in season. If nature is producing them at this time of year, there will be other benefits, such as ideal vitamins and

131

minerals required by the body to stave off winter illnesses.

Others

Nuts and seeds (as well as peanuts, which are actually legumes) are a fantastic source of natural fats, both mono and polyunsaturated. These are great for reducing cholesterol and reduce the risk of heart disease. The fat in these foods also supports your endocrine system (glands), and your organs, including skin.

Consider eating these foods with your protein and fat meals. Avoid eating them with anything sweet or high GI, as fat and sugar together triggers gorge instincts, because nature wants to trick you into putting on weight when you eat this combination –"The Squirrel Formula".

Processed Foods

I've included milk and dairy products in processed foods. It's probably not 100% natural for animals to drink the milk of other mammals, but I cannot say that milk/dairy is unhealthy (unless you're lactose intolerant). Regular milk has the optimal ratio of macronutrients for calves to put on weight and grow muscle, and though calves are quite different physiologically from human beings, there are plenty of healthy nutrients in dairy products suitable for humans.

Dairy products are manufactured from milk and cream. Butters and cheeses are full of saturated fat. Whey is a byproduct of cheese-making (which uses the curds) and is high in protein. Yoghurt is milk that has thickened through the addition of bacteria, and is great for your stomach health.

The advice here is to have natural dairy products in moderation, but be aware that many dairy products have added sugar (such as low-fat yoghurts and flavoured drinks), so keep an eye out for products that are low in fat but contain lots of sugar.

There are many benefits to using butter in your cooking: it is far better than margarine (and tastes better too). Use butter from grass-fed cows, where possible.

Sadly, cheeses with crackers and chutneys trigger the natural instincts to eat more, because of the macronutrient ratios, so only eat on special occasions.

Highly Processed Foods and Fast Foods

You should generally avoid these. However, some processed foods are made from very good ingredients, so check the packaging. Check the content, and examine the ratio of sugar/carbs to protein and fat. If these products are high in carbs and fat, then they are fattening, especially if the ratios tend towards human breast milk. Avoid processed foods with trans fats or hydrogenated fats. Fast food often tastes really good because it appeals to your instincts. Again, the carb/fat ratio sets you into a frenzy and will cause immediate fat deposits.

Sometimes, processed foods can be fine, for example if you are going to do intense training and haven't got some carbs into your system. It may be a good idea to eat something sugary to get your blood sugar ready for a tough cardio session, or replenish your muscles' and liver's sugar stores afterwards. I would sometimes eat jellies or have a sugary drink to replenish, but in moderation. Exercise shouldn't be an excuse to eat these types of foods.

Also, these foods will cause you no harm if you eat them from time to time as a treat, for example a nice little cake in a café once a week, or a chocolate bar or bag of crisps/popcorn at a movie; but if they are part of your everyday routine, you may need to look at it if you wish to really get lean. If you're eating them daily, you may be triggering instincts, which will have you hunting through your cupboards at home late at night.

There are alternative treats you could replace these items with, if you're having them daily, for example a few squares of dark chocolate with a cup of coffee is nice, which will hit the chocolate buzz and is very good for you (don't have the coffee too late in the evening). Maybe a glass of red wine, but watch the sulphites if you have an allergy to them. If you must have a treat, don't deny yourself, but be aware that it may trigger instincts so avoid the combination of high GI carbs and fat, where possible.

The Eat for Winter Diet (How *Not* to Do it)

Definitely not recommended

The following table gives examples of the types of foods people commonly eat, when eating for winter.

Table 5 – Typical Examples of Foods when Eating for Winter

Meal	Examples of Foods Eaten
Breakfast	Toast with butter, pastries with jam/chocolate, donuts, cakes, sugary cereals with fruits, muesli, pancakes, waffles, fatty processed meats, sausage rolls, puddings, sweet yoghurts, juices
Snack	Biscuits, chocolates, crisps, sugary latte/cappucino, juices, fizzy drinks
Lunch	Bread roll/ciabbata/panini/baguette loaded with cheese and sauces with small amounts of meat/salad pasta, pastry pies, creamy mashed potatoes, white rice meals with sauces and fatty meats, cakes/desserts, sugary tea/coffees, fizzy drinks, juices

Snack	Biscuits, chocolate, crisps with sugary tea/coffee, low-fat, high-sugar yoghurts
Dinner	White rice, spaghetti, breads, mash, chips/fries, wedges, burgers, fish in batter, chicken in breadcrumbs, sauces with minimal veg, pizza, ice cream, cakes, sugary and milky tea/coffee, fizzy drink, juices, alcohol
Snack	Popcorn, sweets, chocolates, crisps, flavoured/chocolate/salted nuts, milky tea / coffee, alcohol

In general, the meals outlined are always loaded with *far too many* starchy, energy-dense, low-fibre carb sources for most people with desk jobs.

A Typical Day of Eating for Winter

Following is an example day of eating for winter with an analysis of the day's eating below.

Table 6 – An Example Day of Eating for Winter

Meal	Examples of Foods	Calorie Breakdown
Breakfast 8.00am	Mini fry containing 1 egg, 1 sausage, 1 bacon, 1 pudding, 2 x toast with butter/jam and a cappuccino	**Carbs:** 35g **Protein:** 26g **Fat:** 29g **Calories:** 550
Snack 10.30	2 biscuits and a cappuccino	**Carbs:** 28g **Protein:** 6g **Fat:** 12g **Calories:** 250
Lunch 1pm	Baguette/wrap with breaded chicken,	**Carbs:** 66g **Protein:** 35g

	lettuce, cheese and mayonnaise	**Fat:** 30g **Calories:** 650
Snack 3.30	Brownie and cappuccino	**Carbs:** 47g **Protein:** 8g **Fat:** 25g **Calories:** 450
Dinner 6.30pm	2 baked potatoes, carrots, turnips, 2 pork chops with gravy, bowl of ice cream for dessert	**Carbs:** 88g **Protein:** 34g **Fat:** 13g **Calories:** 600
Snack 9pm	Peanuts, 1 glass of wine	**Carbs:** 42g **Protein:** 9g **Fat:**1.5g **Calories:** 350

Analysis of an Eating for Winter Diet
Total Calories Consumed: 2,750

This is quite a lot of calories and, by far, exceeds what should be consumed by someone with an inactive lifestyle. It could be justified, from a calorific point of view, for an athlete, but not for somebody with a desk job; and even for an athlete, the nutritional support would not be adequate.

Total Carbs Consumed: 310 grams (~1,250 calories)

310 grams of carbs equals about 1,250 calories of energy in essentially sugar form. For an office worker, this could be a surplus of over 400 sugar calories. Add

in a bottle of coke and a fruit juice, and suddenly this figure becomes unworkable for a desk-worker trying to maintain a healthy weight.

Total Fat Consumed: 110 grams (~1,000 calories)

Again, this is a very high amount of fat – well over the recommended daily recommended value. Much of the fat would also have come from hydrogenated fats, which can lead to high cholesterol and poor heart health.

Total Protein Consumed: 120 grams (~500 calories)

This amount of protein is within acceptable parameters, though often such diets do not contain quality, natural products, for example reconstituted meat.

Macronutrient Ratio: 45% carbs/18% protein/37% fat

As well as an excess of calories and low amounts of fibre, the macronutrient ratio has a high-carb and high-fat content, tending towards the ratio found in human breast milk – natures formula to make us put on weight! This explains why these foods make us feel so good while eating them, but why we still want to eat more afterwards. Excess sugar calories will be converted to fat, and fat that is not used by the body for energy and function will also be readily stored as body fat, especially since the body will have sugar spiked with an insulin response six times during the day.

A Note on the 2,000-Calorie Diet

The 2,000-calorie diet is a one-size-fits-all reference diet and has very large margins of error for each macro nutrient. This really is just an average guideline diet, and fails to take into account a person's size, weight, metabolism, gender age, etc. Even the food pyramid does not suit everyone, and is actually in favour of eating for winter, since it tells us to eat mostly carbs every day. A very high-level, endurance athlete might function well on 4,000+ calorie diet, with a lot of carbs present, whereas an inactive, petite person might thrive well on a 1,500-calorie diet. It's all relative, and you must discover what is best for yourself. But, please don't get hung up on calorie counting. Personally, I never do this. I eat when I'm hungry and I try to make the best choice based on what I know will make me feel good afterwards. Once you don't trigger your primal instincts to gorge on autumnal foods, you will be able to hear more clearly what your body needs, rather than overloading these senses with the urge to put on weight for the winter it's programmed to think is coming …

A Note on Carvery/Hotel/Pub Lunches

Often, in carveries, you will see plates piled with starchy carbs such as mashed potatoes, root veg, roast potatoes, chips, fries and/or Yorkshire puddings, along with meat/fish and sauces on top. This amount of carbs would facilitate a six-kilometre + run for a 100-kilogram man. If you're planning on going back to an office desk, reconsider the amount of carbs on your plate. If you eat this quantity of carbs at lunch, and have another large meal in the evening, you would have to be an extremely active person to even have a chance of burning it all off. If the meat is fatty, you will compound the problem in terms of fat storage, given the sugar spike and insulin response you will have caused. Try having less potatoes if you must have them, or avoid them altogether, and load up on root veg like carrots/parsnips/turnip instead (if they are on the menu), which contain plenty of carbs. If low GI veg is on the menu, like broccoli, cauliflower or cabbage, perhaps have small amount of the aforementioned starchy carbs and load up on plenty of this type of veg. Just because everyone else eats a mountain of carbs, it doesn't mean you have to. If you do eat a large quantity of carbs during this meal, for your own sake, please avoid a big dessert too. Often, people eat dessert for the sugar rush to avoid feeling tired immediately after the meal. However, it is because of the huge number of carbs that people suffer from severe mid-afternoon slumps. Stay light, vibrant and full of energy by eating the right number of carbs with your lunch. If I see big chunky veg, I will often ask them to fill up my plate with that, and have the meat/fish too, and I feel fantastic for the entire evening. You don't have to make huge changes immediately: just think about how many carbs you are going to need until later in the evening; make an effort towards minimising that aspect of the meal; and enjoy large quantities of everything else. If you are going back to the forest to chop wood or demolish a house with a lump hammer, then you could consider loading up the plate with the all the starchy carbs, too.

The DEFoW Diet Template

We live in an amazing, privileged, time where our combined ingenuity means that most of us can eat better than the kings and queens of the past. Foods from all seasons are available to us 24/7, 365 days of the year, in supermarkets at very low prices. As stated previously, with this privilege we need to take personal responsibility over the moderation of these foods.

An easy way to think about this moderation daily is to split your day into the four seasons. I tend to start the day with spring for breakfast, summer for lunch, and autumn before and after training for winter, which is a good night's sleep (hibernation). This should be personalised for you, though, because if you are active in the morning due to work or your exercise regime, you may need to shuffle it around a bit.

The following assumes that you work at a desk during normal working day, and are more active in the evenings.

Table 7 – The DEFoW Diet Template

Meal	Objective	Examples of Foods
Breakfast 8am **Season** Spring	Load up on fats and protein here for body function and energy. We want to limit carb intake here to prevent a pronounced insulin spike and keep your body burning fat. The protein will cause a spike, allowing you to absorb nutrients, but the fat will be mobilised for function and energy You should have plenty of carbs from the previous evening to fuel your brain and keep you clear-thinking throughout the morning	Focus on eating protein and fats, eg eggs, meat, fish, nuts, seeds, avocado, and why not throw in some leaves like spinach or rocket for some extra vitamins and minerals Lemon/lime juice in a pint of water Black coffee Drink more water during the morning, too

Lunch 1pm **Season** Summer	You want to start getting some low GI/GL carbs in now for your brain and body, and plenty of fibrous fruit and veg to keep your body healthy In this meal, you also want some lean protein such as turkey, chicken, less-oily fish (eg tuna) or other lean cuts of meat or sources of protein Try to avoid lots of starchy carbs again here, especially in combination with lots of fats, such as mashed potato, baked potato, white rice, etc, with sauces or fatty meats	Lean protein, low GI summer fruit/veg Pint of water Tea/coffee
Mid Afternoon Snack 3.30pm **Season** Late Summer/	You may not feel hungry here, but if you are, snack on some summer fruit/veg here and/or some lean protein If training after work,	Lean protein and controlled, late-summer carbs and a pint of water Potentially add more carbs if training, eg a

143

Early Autumn	it's important to get some carbs in at this point Closer to training, and during training, you could also consider something high GI, if training is intense or heavy; and don't forget hydration	banana, oat, berry and whey protein shake is an option here if training after work. For intense or heavy workout, consider some high GI foods to support, such as sport energy drink with electrolytes, high GI grain product, tubor, fruit or veg, juice etc
Dinner 7.30pm **Season** Autumn	You want to load up on some more protein and carbs here, especially if you've trained in order to maximise your efforts through facilitating recovery. This will ensure a good night's sleep (hibernation); prevent muscle protein breakdown (MPB); and you will have some energy left over for the next morning for your brain and body	A good source of fibrous carb is ideal here, with some more lean protein sources, again with an array of fibrous veg, eg wholegrain rice with mixed veg and chicken, turkey, lean fish Pint of water

Note for Those Who Do Not Exercise: if you are sedentary, you should keep carbs relatively low in all sittings and just give yourself enough for your basic energy needs. If you are naturally slim and have a high metabolism, you have a bit more room to play with here; but for anyone trying to lose weight, really tweak this aspect of your diet downwards to see results.

Note for Those with Manual Jobs: depending on your level of activity, you will need to adjust the amount of carbs in each main meal. You may wish to switch your fat/protein breakfast to later in the day and replace with a carb meal, if your job is physical, so that you have ample energy in the morning for your brain and body. In this case, you could have something like porridge and yoghurt with fruit to start the day, with less fat, and have your fat-based meal in the evening, with fewer carbs at that sitting.

Note for Fitness Enthusiasts/Athletes: if you play sports or take part in physical activity, you should aim to have a moderately sized protein/carb meal a few hours beforehand, to get your body energised and ready; and depending on the intensity/length of the session, you may require a more instant form of sugary food just before, during and after the session. For example, a 500-calorie circuit may require you to have a low-fat, but high-calorie chocolate milk drink, protein and carb shake, or a glucose sports drink with electrolytes to keep your energy levels high and your hydration up during the session. Remember to hydrate well during the day, and ideally have a protein supply ready immediately after training, for example whey. Then, about an hour after training, have your protein/carb meal to prevent muscle break down and encourage muscle maintenance and growth. If you lift weights, or train intensely, you could consider supplementing with fruit juice, creatine and electrolytes before training, to maximise ATP during your session, supplement with BCAAs during training, to encourage muscle growth, and l-glutamine and vitamin and mineral supplements after training, to aid full recovery, and top up anything that may have been depleted due to the stresses on your body, caused by the training. Training hard is trauma that requires ample recovery time and nutrition – the only way to recover is proper diet, hydration and rest. If you do not give your body this support, you may not get the results you deserve for all your hard work!

Sample DEFoW Diet Day

This book is not about telling you specifically what to eat, unlike other diets. It's about giving you the knowledge so that you can choose the right foods to eat for yourself. I prefer the approach of the old proverb: "Give a man a fish and you feed him for a day; teach a man to fish and you feed him for a lifetime." If you can make the right choices based on knowing about your energy requirements, and how your body processes foods and triggers natural instincts, then you should be able to tweak your diet whenever you wish, in order to gain, lose or maintain weight.

You know what *you* like better than anyone else. For example, I like eggs and fried smoked salmon in the mornings, when I have the time; and other days I like protein shakes with peanut butter and/or flax/pumpkin/sunflower seeds blitzed. I'm getting protein and fat from both, and they're delicious. Before a workout, I could have bread and jam with an apple and some cold turkey or chicken on the side or for convenience, sometimes I'll have a banana and raspberry protein shake, which are quick, simple and convenient for me and I really enjoy them. I get fibre, potassium, vitamins and sugar and starch that will give me energy for my training. Often with diets you see complex recipes, the like of which Jamie Oliver would be proud of, and these are fantastic if you have the time to prepare them. However, many of us have very hectic lives, kids to manage, etc, so sometimes this sort of preparation isn't possible, and quick choices need to be made on the run. If you eat what you enjoy, within the parameters outlined, and being mindful of eating varied foods with plenty of colour, fibre, vitamins, carbs, proteins and fats, you will be able to sustain weight and have the energy to deal with the demands of modern life.

In any case, for what it's worth, here is an example of something typical of what I would eat on a sample day.

Table 8 – A Sample Day on The DEFoW Diet

Meal	Examples of Foods	Calorie Breakdown
Breakfast 8am	2 fried eggs and 1-2 grilled rashers of bacon or smoked salmon, nuts and seeds shaken onto the eggs, and perhaps on a bed of rocket/spinach on the side. Pint of water with lemon	**Carb:** 4.3g **Protein:** 26.34g **Fat:** 48.98g **Calories:** 600
Snack 10.30am	You may not be hungry enough to snack at this point but if you are you could have ... An apple or a summer fruit cocktail, eg strawberries, blueberries, raspberries (switching to carbs) and a glass of water	**Carbs:** 17g **Protein:** 0.6g **Fat:** 0.4g **Calories:** 65

	Black coffee/tea rather than milk (small amount of skimmed milk if necessary). If you need sugar keep to minimum	
Lunch 1pm	1-2 lean breast(s) of chicken with broccoli, sweet potato and salad (low-fat dressing, minimise use of oil at this point) and a pint of water	**Carbs:** 55.2g **Protein:** 59.9g **Fat:** 6.4g **Calories:** 530
Snack 3.30pm	You may not be hungry enough to snack at this point but if you are you could have ... Fruit and coffee Pint of water Perhaps supplement with a protein and carb shake before training after work (I like banana and raspberry with natural whey, add oats for extra carb)	**Carbs:** 23.1g **Protein:** 1.1g **Fat:** 0.3g **Calories:** 90
Dinner 7.30pm	Lean steak with onions, mushrooms, carrots, cauliflower and brown rice	**Carbs:** 120g **Protein:** 56g **Fat:** 9g

	Pint of water Glass of red wine or beer (if of legal age), watch the sulphites!	**Calories:** 880

Analysis of DEFoW Diet Sample

Total Carbs: ~200 grams (~800 calories)

For an office worker, this would be the ideal amount of carbs to eat in a day, just enough for the brain and body to function well at rest. If you do exercise a lot, or your job is manual, then you will need to increase this. Also, depending on your body type and metabolism, if you feel *brain fog* or sluggish, then you might want to consider upping the carbs, as required, for your body type/level of energy expenditure.

Total Fat: ~ 65 grams (~600 calories)

This falls within the recommended allowance for fat, and will give you enough fats to support your body's functions. The fats are largely from good sources and so you will feel great and they will improve your health. You will also feel less hungry for a lot of the working day, if eating this type of meal in the morning.

Total Protein Consumed: ~150 grams (~600 calories)

This amount of protein seems quite high, but falls within the recommended allowance and will help keep your body's muscles in good working order. You will also feel fuller for longer.

Macronutrient Ratio: ~40% carbs/~30% protein/ ~30% fat

The macronutrient ratio here has a much more precise amount of energy coming from carb sources. The rest of the energy comes from an equal amount of protein and fat, which, more than just providing instant energy, provide other essential building blocks for the human body.

Please note: this is only a sample, and every day will be different. Moderation and variety are what nature provides us with, so we must mimic that to be as healthy as nature intended.

The natural food sources will also provide plenty of vitamins and minerals to support your body, and the fats will facilitate the absorption of vitamins A, D, E and K.

The timing of foods means that fat storage becomes a more difficult prospect for your body, as you do not have much excess sugar in the first place. Also, the sugar spike will be muted by the fibre in your diet, and if you have a pronounced insulin response, there is little fat present at the same time to be stored off for the future.

Congratulations, You've Just Beaten the System!

Note on Supplementation

If you do supplement with a multivitamin tablet, consider taking it with your fat meal. Vitamins A, D, E and K are fat soluble, whereas the others are water soluble. Having them with a meal containing fat will help to carry them into your system much more efficiently, and they are less likely to just pass through your body.

A Sample Week

Here are some meal ideas based on how I personally eat, but feel free to just follow the template with your own choices. Just remember to consume enough carbs to keep your brain functioning well, but not so much as to cause a surplus of sugar based energy, and thus a pronounced insulin response. Get the rest of your nutrition from fibre, protein and fat sources to keep your body in tip-top condition.

Table 9 – A Sample Week on The DEFoW Diet

Day	Breakfast (Spring)	Lunch (Summer)	Dinner (Autumn)
Monday	1-2 fried eggs (in butter), 1-2 slices bacon, spinach, seeds	Sweet potato and chicken breast with garlic salt and broccoli	Wholegrain rice with scallions abd fresh peas, seasoning and mixed lean meats
Tuesday	1-2 poached eggs, smoked salmon, rocket, walnuts	Lean steak with mushrooms, onions and asparagus with carrots and parsnips	Cajun Chicken breast salad with sliced apple, grapes and brown bread
Wednesday	Avocado with seasoning, nuts and seeds	Turkey breast and broccoli with carrots	Ham and cabbage with moderate potato + skin
Thursday	3-egg omelette with onion, spinach and mixed seeds	Cod baked in lemon juice and balsamic vinegar with sweet potato wedges and mixed leaf salad	Vegetable soup, with spelt bread to dip, lean cuts of meat on side

Friday	1-2 eggs, 1 chop (eg lamb)	Leek and carrot soup with 1-2 slices of spelt bread and lean chicken	Baked tuna steak with brown rice and mixed veg
Saturday	Active day so get carb energy in early ... Porridge with, low-fat greek yoghurt banana, berries and honey (if required)	Then fat-load Chicken and bacon salad with avocado, olive oil and vinegar dressing, topped with mixed seeds and pine nuts	Pork loin with apple sauce and farmhouse vegetable mix
Sunday	Almond, egg, vanilla and cinnamon pancakes, with butter (savoury), or sugar free sauce	Lean roast beef, baby potatoes, broccoli and cauliflower (low-fat sauces)	Some cold lean meat with salad Toasted spelt bread and banana sandwich (avoid butter)

Treats:

We all like our treats now and again. When eating treats again try to utilise the formula. For example, if you're drinking a pint of beer or having a glass of wine, eating nuts with it is more likely to cause fat storage. A low-fat carb snack would be more efficient at this time.

If eating fatty snack try to avoid sugar and carbs, but sometimes you just want to break out. I often go out to a café on the weekends and get myself a peanut butter brownie slice. This is eating for winter and the polar opposite of everything above but boy do I enjoy it with a cup of coffee. It's not a huge cake, but I savour it and enjoy it. I eat it out in the café and it's a bit of an occasion; and I am not at home, even if my instincts are triggered, I tend not to get another, whereas if I had a packet of snacks at home, I would more than likely not have the will power to stop at one. Occasions like Christmas are more difficult to deal with: the best advice here is to not start eating the tin of biscuits by yourself, make sure there are people to share them with ;-)

Why This Works - The FAB Machine

I'm a computer programmer and see the human body as a supercomputer controlling an extremely complex, high-tech and resilient flesh and bone (FAB) machine.

So, let me present to you why exactly this way of eating works so well. Firstly, understand that by eating food, in particular sugary and starchy food, your body's blood sugar levels rise and your body responds by releasing insulin from the pancreas in order for your body to process it (eating protein also causes an insulin response, however, eating carbs generally causes a more pronounced and longer-lasting insulin response). This is why type I diabetics, in particular, need to be so careful with blood sugar levels after eating carbs, as they cannot produce insulin naturally and, as a result, need to inject with adequate insulin to deal with the carbs they've just eaten.

We can learn lessons from diabetics, and everybody needs to be careful about eating too much carb energy, as the body has essentially two modes of operation in terms of energy:

- **Storage Mode:** where you utilise energy from food and absorb excess energy into your body's cells for future use (anabolic).

- **Usage Mode:** where your body uses fat absorbed by your cells when it was in storage mode (catabolic).

When your body has ample sugary fuel for right now in your stomach, seeping into the bloodstream, and your muscle and liver glycogen stores are full, it stands to reason that it will attempt to store as much excess energy as it can for use later on.

It stores sugar in the liver and muscles, and converts excess sugar to fat. It also very easily stores the fat that you've eaten, particularly at the same time as you've eaten carbs, in your fat cells (and it can store literally spoons of fat in one sitting).

Aside: when your body is in storage mode, it is also more likely to build muscle, too, through a process called Muscle Protein Synthesis (MPS), and is less likely to use its own muscles to fuel and repair other parts of the body, such as the brain – a process called Muscle Protein Breakdown (MPB). This will be discussed in more detail later, but essentially, muscles have a dual function, ie to facilitate work, and as a backup battery for the brain in case of starvation.

The sugar in the liver is used to supply other organs, including the brain, when blood sugars are low, and the sugar in muscles is used in case you need to move quickly away from something in order to save yourself. The fat is generally used to provide you with an extremely efficient form of energy for your body when working at a less intense level of activity. Think of sugar as high-octane fuel for afterburners for fight or flight response and power for your brain, and think of fat as diesel, with less acceleration but far more efficiency for covering large distances walking and for surviving for days without food.

As our primary energy source is sugar, it seems that having enough of this results in the insulin response that puts us into this "storage mode". It is no coincidence, then, that this switch is triggered constantly in autumn, when lots of carbs are produced by nature. Traditionally in autumn, we were put into storage mode because of our evolutionary heritage to fatten us up for winter. Unfortunately, now, we are constantly in storage mode because of modern society and all the carb-rich food and sweeties everywhere, so our bodies think that winter is coming all the time.

Here's Why the Diet Works:

1. **Eat protein and fat for breakfast:** this causes a muted insulin response and your body can stay in usage mode (without breaking down muscle because you've eaten protein). Your body will use the fat in the meal for most of its energy and functional requirements. Your brain should have enough glucose from the liver's stores of glycogen, which will have been loaded from the previous evening's carb intake. Your body will also be able to readily use fat from your food and fat cells for resting aerobic energy, but it will use the fat and

protein in the food to support bodily functions also, and so not all those calories can be considered as energy calories. Your appetite will be satisfied all morning.

2. **Eat lean protein and veg for lunch with a small amount of carb:** your body now has been provided with protein and nutrients and some sugar energy for the brain, and this may put you into storage mode. However, because your liver has been used to fuel your brain during the entire morning, it has been depleted somewhat, so the first course of action is to refill that bucket so the blood sugar levels will return to normal quickly. Also, you will have used some glycogen in muscles getting to work and performing basic actions. These stores will also be topped up at this point, which will prevent blood sugar levels spiking too much, thus keeping insulin response to a minimum. If you do eat an excess amount of sugar at this point, it's not the end of the world. Your body will try to convert the excess as fat. However, it takes energy to convert sugar to fat and so less calories will be stored as fat. If you plan on training after work, a carb/protein shake might be a good idea, as a late afternoon snack, to top up muscle glycogen stores and to have sugar and amino acids being supplied

from your stomach during the session for energy and muscle growth and repair.

3. **Eat some carbs and lean meat with veg for dinner:** presuming you have done some exercise after work, your muscles will have been depleted of glycogen again. Your liver will also have been called on to supply energy to the brain and other organs, during the day. Eating carbs now will refill those buckets again, and eating protein with it will provide your body with the amino acids necessary to heal and grow. You will also sleep better and have enough glycogen in your liver to get your brain through the next morning and beyond. During the night, when blood sugars return to normal, you will burn fat as the primary energy source for your resting body, at 85% efficiency!

By eating this way, you will regulate your blood sugar levels, your cells should become less insulin resistant, and you will be burning body fat more readily for most of the day. Of course, a good exercise plan will further accelerate fat loss.

Chapter 6

Getting into Shape

(Lean Gain / Fat Drain)

Make sure the efforts you expend exercising are maximised, and rewarded adequately, by supporting your body with the right nutrition

Getting into Shape

Lean Gain, Fat Drain

It bothers me somewhat when I see training sessions labelled as "fat burning", as this can be misleading. The amount of fat you can burn during resistance training and high intensity-circuit training is minimal, because your body tends to burn sugar during both of these types of sessions, ie anaerobic and high-intensity aerobic exercise.

The only mode where your body really burns fat efficiently is during low-intensity aerobic activity, including resting (think what fuel animals burn when they hibernate: their body fat stores). Animals, including humans, are very efficient at burning fat in a semi-fasted, resting state, ie when blood sugars are normal. The main benefit of training, from a fat-loss perspective, is that you burn more fat than you otherwise would have, while you rest afterwards, as your metabolism is raised for several hours. Furthermore, if you gain lean muscle, your body will burn more calories every day, too.

It is frustrating to see people training very, very hard for months and even years and see very little change in their body shape – no significant increase in muscle mass or decrease in body fat. They train hard enough to see change, but the main problem is nutrition, and in particular, the timing of the correct nutrition, and thus their great efforts are not rewarded as they should be.

This is because:

1. They do not gain lean body mass (ie muscle), because they are not aware of the nutritional requirements to encourage MPS, ie the gaining of new muscle; and to prevent MPB, preventing the body breaking down its own muscle to fuel recovery.

2. They do not lose body fat, because they are constantly eating in a way conducive to fat storage.

Let's deal with building muscle first ...

Every day, we all go through stages of MPS, ie building muscle or being in an anabolic state; and MPB, ie losing muscle or being in a catabolic state. It's subtle during the course of a day and typically, without training, if you eat right you will have a net balance of zero and stay roughly the same. Your body takes its natural shape based on your genetic makeup to the best of its ability, given the food supplied to it. Of course, as you get older, muscle quality and size will reduce due to aging, but resistance training can help fight this and keep the tyre inflated.

For me, aging is the number one reason why everyone should do some form of resistance training, because, in this sense, it is the fountain of youth. Keeping muscles strong and fit means a much better quality of life. A secondary goal is looking well – being in the best shape you can be does wonders for personal confidence.

If your body is going through a strict diet phase, and you have a calorie deficit, and specifically if you do not provide your brain with enough sugar, your body may break down your own muscle to generate glycogen for your brain. Your body can work entirely from fat alone, but the brain requires some glucose, even in a state of ketosis, and so strict diets can actually cause muscle loss as the body cannibalises your muscles, in order to create supplementary fuel for your brain. Extreme examples of this can be seen in photos of people or animals that go through starvation: all muscle and fat are eventually eaten up by the body and brain, in order to survive. The heart and body burns all the fat, and muscle is broken down to supplement the brain's energy requirements. It is interesting that two, major life-giving organs i.e. heart and brain run off fat and sugar respectively, which means they do not readily compete for resources.

Maintaining a positive or negative balance of MPS+MPB will dictate, over a long period, whether you gain or lose muscle. Gaining muscle means remaining in an anabolic state more than a catabolic state, and having the right ingredients available at the right times.

To stay anabolic naturally requires being a lot more clever and disciplined about food timing in conjunction with exercise so that the body can gain significant natural muscle over time. Long-term maintenance of muscle will give you a healthy look and allow you to optimise your genetic heritage well into later life. You will become the best version of yourself for a lot longer. People often say why not just enjoy a shorter life and eat anything you like, but the truth is, for me at least, it wasn't that enjoyable when I was heavy. It's so much more fun now, and I hope it lasts until I am >120 years of age!

Modern research shows that carbs and protein supplementation at the right times can help you stay anabolic. When you train, your body releases hormones to support the MPS cycle (muscle gain), but soon after will start to break down protein again, if the right foods are not present. If the right ingredients are present, your body becomes a muscle-building factory. Protein, in particular the essential amino acids, are very important during and immediately after training, to assist in muscle-building, and carbs can help to spare muscle breakdown.

The main essential amino acid required for MPS is leucine and this is one of the branch chain amino acids (BCAAs for short). It can be found in milk, whey protein or a BCAA supplement. It is also one of the nine essential amino acids, and helps switch on MPS.

Note: It is critical to get this type of protein into your body very soon after an exercise session. Whey is your go-to supply here. If vegetarian, look for something with a good spectrum of essential amino acids, in particular BCAAs.

It is worth noting that, when the body is under stress or sick, glutamine (a non-essential amino acid) can also become depleted, and it is therefore an important supplement after an intense or tough training session, as your body has been compromised, to an extent. Glutamine makes up most of the body's muscle and is used for various other functions, including healing. Even if not training it is a useful supplement to consider, but in the context of intense training, it can assist recovery.

Carbs, on the other hand, help replenish the body's glycogen stores, which are also reduced after training. Replenishing these leads to more recovery, and insulin presence can retard muscle protein breakdown. Studies have shown that whey protein causes enough of an insulin spike to assist with MPS and retard MPB, but if the training was intense, the recovery period will be longer, and when insulin has returned to normal levels, MPB may ensue. Therefore, a low GI autumnal carb source, after training, could assist with keeping the body anabolic for longer, and having lean protein at the ready with it, for example brown rice or bread with turkey, chicken breast or tuna, etc, will provide the body with the slow release of sugar energy and the amino acids necessary over a longer period. This, in turn, will ensure that you stay anabolic and thus recover better and maintain and add a little bit of new muscle each day.

Here is my suggestion regarding nutrition around a training session:

Three Hours before Training: your regular meal with some carbs and protein present.

Approximately One Hour Pre-training: a carb source with protein and lots of water.

I might have a whey protein shake with banana, berries, juice *or* maybe even bread, jam and an apple or other fruit with protein milk, etc.

Before high-intensity training, it might be worth loading up on sugar, depending on the job at hand. If it's a long session, more slow burn carbs, like oats, are good. If it's really long endurance work, some fat could be added.

Creatine is something else to consider pre-training, as it can help yield more explosive strength during your session. Creatine supports the ATP energy system and may help you perform a little better if you are fully hydrated and fuelled up with electrolytes and carbs.

During Training: carb up with protein, in particular leucine (contained in milk, or BCAA supplement).

Personally, my go-to here is chocolate milk during a hypertrophy (strength-building) period. It's low in fat, high in carbs, and contains milk protein. It also contains natural electrolytes, so ticks many boxes for exercise. Don't overdo it, however, as even though it is low in fat, for example 2%, over 500 mililitres, that's 10 grams of fat consumed, along with a lot of carbs. If I wished to drop body fat, I would replace this with BCAAs mixed with juice and water.

Within an Hour after Training: immediately after training, take whey protein, to encourage MPS.

If feeling very depleted, I might occasionally eat sweets, such as jellies, or take a glucose drink at this time to replenish glycogen stores. However, if I've had a large portion of chocolate milk during training, this may not be necessary and, as stated, it's important not to overdo it.

Sometimes, after intense exercise L-glutamine supplementation can be helpful for recovery. Also, a good multivitamin tablet and proper hydration with electrolytes will also assist here.

One to Two Hours after Training: a good high fibre, low GI carb meal with lean natural protein, for example brown rice, bread, wheat along with chicken, turkey, or other lean meat or fish.

Now Let's Deal with Burning Fat ...

So, with all the carbs outlined above, you might be worried about depositing fat. You need to carefully consider the carb intake, based on the type of training you undertake, and get the balance right. It's pretty easy to work out, with a Smartphone app or an online calculator, the amount of calories burned up during exercise. It's a bit more difficult with weight training to gauge calories expended, so a little bit of trial and error might be needed to get it right. Some tools for this are linked to at following URL:

www.donteatforwinter.com/book-links

A relatively tough half-hour session might burn 250 calories, which would equate to 50 grams of carbs, evenly distributed over an hour. A smoothie with a banana and portion of oats would cover the calories burned during the session, if taken before the session. A tough spinning class might burn 400 calories, and so the requirement is larger for this type of session. With weights, there is more muscle protein synthesis, so a greater amount for protein and slow-burn carbs a couple of hours later will keep the body from breaking down protein.

This is where the precise carb control comes in – you just need enough to fuel and recover, above and beyond your normal daily requirements.

In terms of burning fat, then, I would tend to refrain from eating many carbs in the morning and stick to the Don't Eat for Winter guidelines. I focus on getting my fats in during the first few hours of the day, especially if I train in the evening (an adjustment would be required for those training during the day, or in the morning). In this scenario, my brain will do fine based on the carbs I ate the night before, and my body will run off the fat I eat and my fat reserves. The protein in my breakfast should protect against muscle-protein breakdown, and my body will use the fat for energy and body function, rather than storing it, as my blood sugar level and thus my insulin response is controlled. I'll also feel full all morning, because fat and protein are more satiating.

If you train in the mornings, flip the whole thing and load up on carbs first thing. Oats with fat-free yoghurt, berries, honey, etc is a good choice here, and your lunch could also contain carbs and protein (perhaps more early summer stuff). You could have eggs and fish/meat for an evening meal, with some low GI veg or salad to maximise fat burning during the night.

For those who train in the evening, a template for the day might look like the following:

Breakfast: protein and fat, for example avocado, nuts, seeds, eggs, meat, oily fish. Throw in salad for greens.

My go-to is eggs and bacon rashers, turkey rashers or fried smoked salmon. Often, I scatter my eggs with pumpkin, sunflower and other mixed seeds for extra nutrients. Some days, I make almond and egg pancakes and eat them with butter – a nice savoury snack – and on other days, I might have an avocado with walnuts. If in a hurry, a flax seed or peanut butter protein shake can also do the trick (just keep the carbs low).

Snack: if I feel like my brain is foggy, I could have some fresh fruit, or if very hungry, which is rare, some nuts.

Lunch: veg, salad and fish/meat. Start getting carbs from veg.

One Hour before Training: carb and protein snack, for example an apple and a jam sandwich (hold the fat) with a protein shake *or* a banana, whey and creatine smoothie.

If intense training, potentially, load up on more sugar closer to training.

During Training: chocolate milk if not concerned about weight gain, otherwise, juice and water drink with BCAAs.

Water always, or electrolyte drink if a sweaty session.

Immediately after training: whey protein shake: add something sweet, if feeling particularly depleted of energy, and l-glutamine if very fatigued. Hydration and multivitamins are no harm either, at this time.

Dinner One to Two Hours after Training: low GI carbs (whole grains and veg) and lean meat (turkey, chicken, tuna, or other lean cuts).

Instructors in gyms should always advise their students in this capacity. They would see a huge change in their members by helping them get their diet tweaked, and see much better results, which would result in the gym getting a great reputation, as results speak for themselves.

Now that you have some more knowledge, you can apply it to get those lean gains. This will give you the look you are after, and make you more functional, less prone to injury and feel generally healthier and more confident.

Everything I've done to tweak my diet is laid out above, and I've achieved excellent results from eating like this. I hope it works just as well, if not better, for you!

Remember to hydrate with every meal, and if you have a particularly sweaty session, or you're prone to sweating a lot, invest in some electrolyte tablets and have them ready for when you need them. This will help you keep your concentration, facilitate better muscle contractions, and help you to avoid cramp.

Getting Fit v Getting in Shape

The only way to lose fat effectively is through food awareness. However, a good exercise plan can accelerate your fat loss considerably. This is primarily because you burn calories while exercising, but also because you raise your metabolism when recovering after exercise. When exercising, you typically burn sugar, which in turn lowers blood sugar levels. This will keep you, or put you into, energy usage mode, as opposed to energy storage mode.

There's a subtle difference between getting fit and getting in shape, but they are not mutually exclusive. You can be strong, cardio fit, have endurance, flexibility and good coordination and also be overweight. You might not be capable of four-minute kilometres over a 10-kilometre run with 40% body fat, but that is down to the amount of energy required to move all that extra weight for each stride. Being fit could mean choosing to be heavier for your sport, to gain advantage.

Getting Fit: can be interpreted in many ways, but essentially it means working one or more of your fitness systems to improve your capacity, efficiency, agility and skill, over time.

Getting in Shape: is more aesthetic in nature, and generally means developing lean muscle mass and losing body fat, so that you become the ideal version of your physical self.

Either way, exercise is absolutely necessary to keep you strong and healthy, so that you can deal with life's challenges, and looking good too. A fit body also leads to a fit mind so let's deal with fitness, before we deal with getting in shape.

There are various types of fitness, and athletes need to draw on some or all of these systems. We can learn from them in order to tailor training for our individual needs, so as to get fit and in better shape, depending on our goals:

1. **Explosive strength:** power and speed, utilising the anaerobic systems.
2. **Intense cardio:** maximum effort, utilising both anaerobic and aerobic systems.
3. **Endurance cardio:** long distance/duration, utilising primarily aerobic systems.
4. **Suppleness, mobility and flexibility:** body agility, utilising tendons, joints and muscles.
5. **Coordination:** skilfulness, utilising mind and body motor control.
6. **Body composition:** not really a fitness, but all of the above can play a part, along with diet.

Explosive Strength: is generated from what is known as your fast-twitch muscle fibres (typically bigger stronger looking muscles like that of a sprinter) loaded with ATP (muscle contraction energy) and glycogen (sugar stored in muscles). This is generally anaerobic in nature, because you don't need oxygen to perform actions. Of course, if you try do anything at speed for long enough, you will then move into your aerobic/cardiovascular zone and start training that. Typical athletes who train these systems are sprinters, fighters, shot-putters, etc, Olympic weight lifters and power lifters. The primary fuel required for these sports is sugar preloaded into the body.

Intensive Cardio: intense cardio exercise, such as circuit training, boxing, cycling at pace, and fast running beyond short sprints, all use up sugars in blood mixed with oxygen, which undergo chemical reactions to produce ATP in order for your muscles to contract. It is called aerobic exercise, because it makes you breath hard in order to take in more oxygen. This sort of exercise will raise your heart rate and intensify breathing, in order for oxygenated blood to be pumped around your body so that chemical reactions can occur with carb (sugar) fuel, primarily, and thus power your muscles. This can be a very tough type of exercise for athletes, as overworking this system means that the body cannot produce energy fast enough, and leads to the creation of nasty byproducts, which make the exercise very painful and quick recovery difficult. It invokes a combination of slow and fast twitch muscle fibres. Examples of athletes who train this system are short- distance runners, rowers, kettlebell athletes, and boxers.

Endurance Cardio: this type of fitness is for athletes who need to work with an elevated heart rate for a long time. Heart rate is kept below maximum so that the body can produce enough ATP to keep the athlete going at a certain pace, potentially for hours. This activity involves burning a combination of sugar and fat with the oxygen in your blood and invoking mostly slow-twitch muscle fibres (think of a slender long-distance athlete), primarily for contractions. Typical athletes here would include marathon runners, long-distance cyclists, swimmers and triathletes. There are other fitness aspects involved here, such as the ability to withstand inflammation in joints and tendons, and general toughness. This type of fitness comes only with endless hours of training.

Suppleness, Mobility and Flexibility: this type of fitness involves having good mobility, flexible hamstrings, groin, back and shoulders, and having all the tendons and muscles knot-free, and joints working well. It also means having a good strong core (muscles in mid-section, front, back and sides) to assist with posture and movement. Typical athletes with this sort of fitness are yoga practitioners, martial artists and gymnasts.

Coordination: this sort of fitness involves more of a link between the mind and body – an elevated level of motor-control skills to make your body do what you want it to do exactly when you want to do it. In other words, timing and skill. A person is often born with a greater talent in this area and if developed they can often do what seems amazing or even impossible to others. Swinging at something, playing a musical instrument, throwing something at a target, and kicking something with accuracy all involve timing and skill, with the mind and body working as a unit. An increase of this type of skill can be developed with practice. Typical athletes who use this system include golfers, hurlers, darts-players, drummers (yes they are athletes), snooker-players, bowlers, soccer-players, goal-keepers, ice-skaters, baseball-players, etc.

Body Composition: this is not necessarily a fitness, but getting this right can make you better suited to your chosen sport. Some athletes need to be heavy, for example sumo wrestlers and tug-of-war specialists; some need very low body fat, for example rock climbers and gymnasts; and others need to be loaded with muscle mass, for example power lifters and rugby players. It is the art or science of eating and training correctly for your sport, in order to get your body into optimal condition for the task at hand, and it takes a lot of planning and refining.

Many athletes need to utilise all of the above systems. The best example I can think of is someone like Conor McGregor, who needs explosive power for knockout punches; fast cardio for a flurry of punches and kicks over a five-minute round; endurance cardio fitness for lasting the distance over many rounds; suppleness, mobility and flexibility for static strength, agility, high kicks, lock holds, and being able to deal with being contorted by an opponent, when being held in a particular hold; coordination for accuracy, nimbleness and avoiding blows; and of course body composition to get into a weight division, with the correct ratio of muscle, fat and water.

The fitness types outlined above are available for everyone to train, but each individual needs to think about their goals, and train/eat according to these. Essentially, we are all closet athletes and our bodies are capable of amazing things and will adapt to almost anything you throw at it given time; but, you must train and eat for each activity in a different way, and with a good level of consistency.

Every athlete will have a specific meal plan in place to assist with both their training activities and recovery. For example:

- To support explosive power an athlete will need carbs in the form of glycogen stored in their muscles and more in their blood/stomach to keep refilling. They will also require protein for muscle growth and recovery.
- To support intense cardio, an athlete will require lots of high GI carbs to get glycogen into their muscles and liver fast, and have a readily available

supply in their bloodstream, feeding muscles during exercise.

- To support endurance, an athlete will need lots of lower-GI carbs and fats to get them through a long day of activity. They will also potentially burn some of their body's fat stores during a race, so it's important to have a healthy amount of fat on the body, but not so much as to negatively affect performance. These athletes will typically need to be hydrating with electrolytes and supplementing fuel during and after exercise.
- Athletes who are supple need a good diet to support their muscles, tendons and joints. Plenty of good fats/oils and protein will keep the body mobile and keep muscles strong.
- Athletes who require coordination must often concentrate over hours and hours. The main fuel for the brain is also glucose, so blood sugars should be kept stable with lower-GI carb sources. Other items like caffeine can help these athletes keep their focus.
- Athletes who focus on body composition need to get their macronutrient ratio and food volume right. This means finding a formula for how much protein, fat and carbs they should eat for their ideal body type, and time them correctly around their activities.

All athletes should ensure that they are hydrated and get a full spectrum of minerals and vitamins from their diet/supplementation.

In terms of an average person, there is a lot to learn from all these types of activities – perhaps there is a need for a bit of everything. The common factor, really, is having the correct amount of fuel and nutrients for your body for the task at hand. You have specific requirements for your work and level of activity, and should make it your business to find out exactly those needs.

If your goal is simply to get into clothes, it is basically 80% diet. Yes, you will burn more fat at rest after you exercise, but if you eat too much of the wrong food you will never lose weight. If you want to be able to play more with your kids or dance all night, then you need to be cardio fit; if you wish to climb mountains, you need endurance and low body fat; if you wish look really athletic and muscular in your swim suit, then you need to work on explosive strength and body composition. All these activities need to be supported with the right foods.

In my experience, most people want the following:

- To look good in (and out) of clothes.

- To be a bit more cardio fit for use in everyday life.
- To be more supple, to reduce risk of injury or levels or pain.

To Look Good: this requires two main focuses: resistance/explosive training and diet. Diet is the most important aspect, but resistance training will do two things: improve your muscle quality, shape, definition, and increase your metabolism after training so that you are burning more fat when you are resting. When doing this sort of training, it is important to have enough carbs available to you during training, and plenty of protein to assist with recovery afterwards. You don't need to load up on carbs and eat for a marathon for this type of exercise: just eat enough so that you are not light-headed or yawning. If you are breathing too hard doing this sort of exercise, you are using your aerobic system, which isn't the goal. Yes, you will start breathing after reps, but you do not need to go overboard. In my experience, circuit training does not achieve the same physical results as weight training, with longer rest periods so that exercises are performed correctly through full range of motion. Weight training will make your muscles more aesthetic, and you get the metabolism rising/fat-burning effects afterwards too. Don't be afraid of the effort – enjoy it! You are designed to work in this way, and you will feel good from the endorphins released.

More cardio fit: in order to get more cardio fit, you need to push your heart rate up but you must eat right for this. You could go for 30-45-minute run, do a circuit class, spinning class, play a game of five-a-side, squash or whatever. The only way to eat right for this is to have enough sugar in your system for the activity at hand. Eating a sandwich 20 minutes before training won't do it: if eating slow release carbs, you should eat them in good time before the session. However, I would suggest having some sort of higher-GI food, such as ripe fruit before this type of training. This sort of exercise won't really help with fat loss during the exercise itself, because the chemical reactions required are too demanding to utilise your fat-burning energy exclusively. However, not all is lost, as your metabolism will be elevated for a long time afterwards, and so you will burn more fat than you otherwise would have when you rest. Your overall fitness will also improve greatly. It is important also to be well hydrated for this type of training, and to eat adequate protein for repair.

To assist with weight loss, hour-long, slow cardio activities a good distance from your meals will help. Slow jogging, fast walking, hiking (not pushing it), leisurely cycles, etc, would all assist here. Keep heart rate low enough that you are able to talk all the way through the exercises, and hydrate well.

To Be More Supple: this sort of training is probably the most enjoyable and relaxing, but is still very demanding, and will help tone up muscle and improve posture. It involves lots of static holds, stretches, mobility exercises, etc. A good yoga class is a typical example of this type of training. Eating for this sort of exercise means a good balanced diet of vitamins, minerals, fats, proteins and carbs. You will need some carbs for static holds, protein for repair work after stretches, and fats to support joints, etc. If you want a nice shapely waist and six-pack, it can be achieved through lots of core work. But again, eating must be controlled to reveal the fruits of your labour.

A suggested work out plan each week, with all of these goals in mind, might look like something like this:

Table 10 – Suggested Exercise Plan

Day	Exercise	Food Focus
Mon	Upper body weight training session with focus on body parts you wish to improve, for example chest, back, shoulders, arms and core	Make sure you have adequate protein, and some carbs to have enough energy for training. Don't overdo it with the carbs: be precise

Tue	Light cardio, 45 minutes, approximately, for example a long-recovery jog/walk	Keep carbs relatively low to burn more fat, and hydrate well
Wed	Yoga or other core strength- and stretching-based routine, for example Pilates	Eat a very balanced diet today, don't overdo carbs, use protein to recover and hydrate well
Thur	Fast cardio, circuit training, soccer, squash, sprints, boxing MMA	For this exercise, you need a good amount of sugar in your blood. You won't burn much fat while exercising, as you are training high intensity cardio fitness. Push too hard here, without adequate energy, and you won't feel right. Hydrate well, as always
Fri	Weight training session with focus on the body parts you wish to improve. If you did upper body on Monday, you might want to focus on glutes and legs today (quads, calves and hamstrings), finish with core	Make sure you have adequate protein, and enough carbs to fill your glycogen stores and keep them topped up, in order to have enough energy for training
Sat	Light cardio, on hour+ on a long recovery run/walk	Keep carbs controlled to burn more fat, but fuel up on Low GI carbs to keep you going strong for the duration of the

		session. and hydrate very well. For long duration exercise bring snacks to refuel
Sun	The religious guys were right – you need a day of rest, but get out with family/friends for a light walk even and use your fitness to have fun!	Get yourself a coffee and a treat. You deserve it!

For each session, you should always hydrate well with mineral water and no added chemicals (I personally avoid tap water unless I have no other choice). Sugary glucose drinks are sometimes advertised as hydrating with electrolytes, but they often don't contain the full spectrum. Check labels and look for a complete set of electrolytes or get a supplement and make your own. Glucose drinks can be helpful during fast cardio sessions, but in general they will cause a pronounced insulin response which will inhibit fat-burning, and are not necessary for most low-intensity sessions. It could be better here to make your own simple electrolyte drink from an electrolyte supplement, with lemon juice and water, and customise the amount of sugar, depending on the intensity of the workout. If you are an athlete, you will need to get very precise about your carb intake, and timing of same.

Chapter 7

Conclusion

(Baby Steps)

Don't bite off more than you can chew, change habits one by one. A tiny change now results in immense changes over time.

Conclusion

The Little Voice

I think everyone has the little voice (TLV) in their head that persuades them to perform some action against their better judgement. It's not some evil demon bidding that them to do its will (at least I hope not), but it might be their subconscious instincts constructing thoughts in order to persuade their conscious mind to take action.

In the case of food, here's how the internal conversations go for me:

Me: "No, I won't eat that chocolate."

TLV: "Go on, just one won't make any difference."

Me: "Ok, I'll have just one – just to taste them. Yum!"

[Silence for a minute]

TLV: "Maybe you should have one more???"

Me: "No, I shouldn't have even eaten the first one!!!"

TLV: "But that last one was so tasty, one more won't make a difference…"

Me: "I shouldn't."

TLV: "Go on, just one more? Then I'll leave you alone."

Me: "OK, one more and that's it and I mean it!"

TLV: "OK sure thing ☺"

[Silence]

TLV: "It's me again, fancy one more???"

Me: "No, no, no. I've already overdone it."

TLV: "But you haven't tried the praline ones yet. Just try one of them – they're really nice, I'd say."

Me: "Yeah, just a praline; just to taste them."

[Silence]

TLV: "And what about the soft toffee one? Surely we gotta try that one too."

Me: "OK, OK. I'll try that too."

TLV: "That's the spirit."

Me: "Ah, look there's only one left, might as well eat it now too and they'll be gone..."

Me: *Twiddles thumbs*

Me: "I NEED MORE CHOCOLATES!!!"

Me: *Searches house for 30 minutes for more goodies*

Me: "I feel disgusting – another day of my diet ruined!!!"

TLV: [Total silence]

– Ends –

Don't feel guilty about this sort of inner dialogue. You're not weak and you should not feel bad for giving in. You should understand that these are powerful natural processes that have been invoked once that first chocolate is eaten. Your body will insist that you eat more because it has received information that suggests winter is coming, and it is trying to protect you by triggering thoughts to make you eat more, even though your conscious mind knows better. It's a battle between your conscious mind and your subconscious instincts, and the only way to win the war, is to understand it. My advice on this matter is not to eat the first chocolate, or whatever it is you are being tempted to eat, unless you are prepared to be pestered by "the little voice".

It is okay to sometimes indulge – but do it consciously. I go for a little treat most Saturdays, and I really, really enjoy it. Every time, the minute I eat it, I want another; but I know it's just the little voice. I'm also in a café, so it's more difficult for me to go and buy another than if I were at home with a packet of cookies or cakes. I also have to travel a distance to get it, so there are barriers in place and effort involved in getting it that my instincts have difficulty overcoming.

I look forward to it, enjoy it, and once the voice subsides, I feel good about myself because I had a delicious treat, which was very enjoyable, and I managed to overcome the voice by making it difficult to gorge.

I'm not going to lie to you: sometimes the voice wins. We all have those moments, but I don't beat myself up over it anymore. I just go back to the Don't Eat for Winter guidelines as soon as I can. Generally, I'm totally satisfied with my food and am never hungry, and really feel good when I don't overdo it on the autumnal starches and sugars. By eating this way, typically, I settle back down to my natural weight.

Old Habits Die a Long, Slow, Painful Death

If you try to break a habit quickly, it can be difficult. Sometimes going cold turkey is just too much, and then there's a rebound because you miss terribly, what you've "given up". Giving up something means it was important to you, otherwise you wouldn't be giving it up. So, how do you break habits? You don't! You change them!

Look at everything you eat during the day, and on day one make a tiny change, for example take half a spoon less of sugar in your cappuccino. After a little while, you'll wonder how you could have had it that sweet before! If you have two slices of toast for brekkie, try one, and add in an egg, some meat, for example bacon, salmon, turkey or other protein/fat source instead.

It's little changes over a long period that make the biggest difference. For example, if you had three cups of tea/coffee a day with a level-teaspoon less sugar in each; this one simple tweak would equate to removing almost *five-and-a-half kilograms* of sugar from your diet over the course of a year.

Continue this approach with everything. By doing this, I've gone from milky lattes with spoons of sugar, to black coffee with no sugar. I couldn't have dreamt of that a few years ago, but I didn't feel the transition because I changed slowly, and now I drink black coffee with meals and it's just as enjoyable as the sweet lattes once were.

It's the same with training, don't try and run without walking, or perform an intense circuit without first breaking your muscles in gently. The muscle soreness may put you off and you need not do that to yourself. Give your body and mind a chance to adapt over the correct amount of time and the results will astound you as there are literally no limits to what you can achieve when you train and don't strain.

Control Your Carbs

This key to this whole book can be summarised as follows: **Control the sugar energy your body receives by limiting the number of carbs you eat daily based on your energy requirements; and avoid eating carbs and fat at the same time where possible.**

Remember, an excess of sugar energy will cause fat storage, and to make matters worse, if you eat fat at the same sitting, your body will store it more readily because the insulin response tells your cells to receive sugar and fat. This type of food tastes really good, because it typically appears in autumn, and triggers our natural survival instincts, which fool us into stuffing our faces. This is how we evolved and adapted to be efficient at putting on weight in order to survive the cold, bleak winter ahead. Before the modern era, once that food was gone, we would burn off the excess weight during the winter months, as food became more scarce. Today, that food scarcity never happens, so chronic weight gain is the result, and many people end up with serious health and self-esteem issues, through no fault of their own. The game was rigged, and the cards are still stacked against us, however, things have changed for us because now we know better, and are no longer ignorant to the facts. It's GAME OVER for fat.

We now know that low-fat/high-carb diets are no longer the way to go, and that science and its orthodox following propagated the wrong "facts" and led us astray for far too long. We now understand that commercial entities prey on our instincts, relying on our impulse purchases to gain profit. All the evidence points to lower-carb diets, with adequate amounts of fat and protein being better for us. The carbs that you do eat should be "good carbs", ie natural, fibrous, nutritious, slow-burning, low GI carbs, and eaten daily along with healthy sources of protein and fat. They should come from as many sources as possible, and in their natural form, in order not only to fuel our bodies with the energy and protein we need, but also to supply us with fibre and all the essential vitamins and minerals necessary so that we look and feel our best.

When eating meals think of the energy food as the focus of the meal, and what you should eat with it, ie:

- When eating a carb loaded meal, tend toward having less fat at the same sitting (and lean protein)
- When eating a fat loaded meal, tend towards having less carbs with that meal (and any protein)

If you do all of this over time you will become the improved version of you.

Finally, you should be active and have fun. Get out into nature and enjoy sunshine and good air. Combine resistance training with cardio and flexibility work, and support this training with diet and adequate rest. Don't be a hero and do too much too soon: be smart, work hard and use exercise as a social outlet to surround yourself with like-minded, supportive people. If you see others doing well, compliment them and ask them about their journey, too. We are all in this together.

I want to personally thank you for reading my book. I hope you got something from it and I wish you the very best with your weight loss. I fought with mine for many years and found it very difficult to control, even though I trained hard, until I discovered that eating for winter, all the time, was the root cause of my problem. Now, when I *Don't Eat for Winter*, I drop to my ideal weight quickly, and it's easily maintained.

I enjoy every bit of food that I eat: I savour it and I relish how I feel afterwards. I get rewarded with my performance in the gym and from people when they say I look well. You really are a worthwhile project and have an amazing, resilient, FAB machine at your disposal, that has survived millions of years of adaptation to extremely tough environments. It's eagerly waiting for you give it what it needs to thrive so remember –

Don't Eat for Winter

– at least not all the time, in order to reveal your true body – the body nature intended you to have.

If you have applied the rules of The DEFoW Diet to your life and you wish to share your success story with us, please do so here:

www.donteatforwinter.com/testimonials

Reference List

Adams, S. (2012). Obesity killing three times as many as malnutrition. Telegraph.co.uk. Retrieved 3 January 2017, from http://www.telegraph.co.uk/news/health/news/9742960/Obesity-killing-three-times-as-many-as-malnutrition.html

Bao, J., Atkinson, F., Petocz, P., Willett, W., & Brand-Miller, J. (2011). Prediction of postprandial glycemia and insulinemia in lean, young, healthy adults: glycemic load compared with carbohydrate content alone. *American Journal of Clinical Nutrition*, 93(5), 984-996. doi:10.3945/ajcn.110.005033

Berg J.M., Tymoczko J.L., & Stryer, L. *Biochemistry*. 5th edition. New York: W H Freeman; 2002. Section 30.2, Each organ has a unique metabolic profile. Available from: https://www.ncbi.nlm.nih.gov/books/NBK22436/

Brannigan et al. (2009). Hypothermia is a significant medical risk of mass participation long-distance open water swimming. *Wilderness & Environmental Medicine*, 20(1), 14-18. http://dx.doi.org/10.1580/08-WEME-OR-214.1

Choi A. et al. (2015). Association of lifetime exposure to fluoride and cognitive functions in Chinese children: A pilot study, *Neurotoxicology and Teratology*, 47, 96-101. http://dx.doi.org/10.1016/j.ntt.2014.11.001

Davilla, D. Food and Sleep. (2017). Sleepfoundation.org. Retrieved 10 January 2017, from https://sleepfoundation.org/sleep-topics/food-and-sleep

Eaton, S. B., Shostak, M., & Konner, M. (1988). *The Paleolithic prescription: a program of diet & exercise and a design for living*. New York: Harper & Row.

Ebbeling C.B., Swain, J.F., Feldman, H.A., Wong, W.W., Hachey, D.L., Garcia-Lago, E., & Ludwig, D.S. (2012). Effects of dietary composition on energy expenditure during weight-loss maintenance. *JAMA*. 307(24), 2627-2634. doi:10.1001/jama.2012.6607

Public Health England (2015). E-cigarettes: an evidence update. Retrieved 10 January 2017, from https://www.gov.uk/government/publications/e-cigarettes-an-evidence-update

Ezzati et al. (2012-2014). Global and regional mortality from 235 causes of death for 20 age groups in 1990 and 2010: A systematic analysis for the Global Burden of Disease Study 2010, *The Lancet*, 380(9859), 2095-2128. http://dx.doi.org/10.1016/S0140-6736(12)61728-0.

Fats 101. (2017). American Heart Association. Heart.org. Retrieved 9 January 2017, from http://www.heart.org/HEARTORG/HealthyLiving/FatsAndOils/Fats-101_UCM_304494_Article.jsp#.WHLjwVWLTIW

Freudenrich, C. (2000). How Fat Cells Work. HowStuffWorks.com. Retrieved 3 January 2017, from http://science.howstuffworks.com/life/cellular-microscopic/fat-cell.htm

Gunnars, K. (2013). 23 studies on low-carb and low-fat diets – time to retire the fad. *Authority Nutrition*. Retrieved 3 January 2017, from https://authoritynutrition.com/23-studies-on-low-carb-and-low-fat-diets/

Jamieson, S. (2016). Britain's squirrels are getting fat thanks to the warm winter . Telegraph.co.uk. Retrieved 5 January 2017, from http://www.telegraph.co.uk/news/earth/wildlife/12084226/Britains-squirrels-are-getting-fat-thanks-to-the-warm-winter.html

Kearns C.E., Schmidt, L.A.,& Glantz, S.A. (2016). Sugar industry and coronary heart disease research: A historical analysis of internal industry documents. *JAMA Intern Med*. 176(11), 1680-1685. doi:10.1001/jamainternmed.2016.5394 http://jamanetwork.com/journals/jamainternalmedicine/article-abstract/2548255

Lennerz, B., Alsop, D., Holsen, L., Stern, E., Rojas, R., & Ebbeling, C. et al. (2013). Effects of dietary glycemic index on brain regions related to reward and craving in men. *American Journal Of Clinical Nutrition*, 98(3), 641-647. doi:10.3945/ajcn.113.064113

Martin, L. J. et al. (2016). Dietary fats explained: *Medline Plus Medical Encyclopedia*. Medlineplus.gov. Retrieved 9 January 2017, from https://medlineplus.gov/ency/patientinstructions/000104.htm

Mayo Clinic Staff. Counting calories: Get back to weight-loss basics. Mayo Clinic, 2017, Retrieved 5 January 2017, from http://www.mayoclinic.org/healthy-lifestyle/weight-loss/in-depth/calories/art-20048065

Mooney, A. (2013). Addicted to ... Food? Harvard Medical School. Hms.harvard.edu. Retrieved 5 January 2017, from https://hms.harvard.edu/news/addicted-food-7-3-13

Neel, James, V. (1962). Diabetes mellitus: A "thrifty" genotype rendered detrimental by "progress"? *American Journal of Human Genetics*.14(4), 353-362. https://www.ncbi.nlm.nih.gov/pmc/articles/PMC1932342/

Neel, James, V. "The "thrifty genotype" in 1998. (2014). *Nutrition Reviews,* 57(5) 2009, 2-9. http://nutritionreviews.oxfordjournals.org/content/57/5/2

O'Connor, Anahad (2016). How the sugar industry shifted blame to fat. Nytimes.Com, 2016, http://www.nytimes.com/2016/09/13/well/eat/how-the-sugar-industry-shifted-blame-to-fat.html?_r=2

Voegtlin, W. L. (1975). *The stone age diet: Based on in-depth studies of human ecology and the diet of man*. New York: Vantage Press.

Wax, E. et al. (2017). Protein in diet. *MedlinePlus Medical Encyclopedia*. Medlineplus.gov. Retrieved 10 January 2017, from https://medlineplus.gov/ency/article/002467.htm

Wikipedia: Thrifty gene hypothesis. (2017). En.wikipedia.org. Retrieved 3 January 2017, from https://en.wikipedia.org/wiki/Thrifty_gene_hypothesis

Visit www.donteatforwinter.com/references for updates/additions to this section and for more interesting links.

Printed in Poland
by Amazon Fulfillment
Poland Sp. z o.o., Wrocław